Medication
Safety
and
Cost
Recovery

A Four-Step

Approach

for Executives

Chip Caldwell
Charles Denham, M.D.

Foreword by
Lucian L. Leape, M.D.

ACHE Management Series

Health Administration Press

Medication

Safety

and

Cost

Recovery

A Four-Step

Approach

for Executives

05   04   03   02   01   5   4   3   2   1

Library of Congress Cataloging-in-Publication Data

Caldwell, Chip.
    Medication safety and cost recovery: a four-step approach for executives/
    by Chip Caldwell and Charles Denham.
        p. cm.
    Includes bibliographical references and index.
    ISBN 1-56793-154-5
    1. Medication errors. I. Denham, Charles. II. Title.
    RM146 .C354 2001
    362.1′782—dc21   2001024388
                                                                  CIP

The paper used in this publication meets the minimum requirements of American National Standard for Information Sciences-Permanence of Paper for Printed Library Materials, ANSI Z39.48-1984. ∞ ™

Project manager: Cami Cacciatore; Book design: Matt Avery;
Cover design: Jason Ackley

Health Administration Press
A division of the Foundation of the
    American College of Healthcare Executives
1 North Franklin Street, Suite 1700
Chicago, IL 60606-3491
(312) 424-2800

To Ben Latimer,
the inspiration for this book,
who consistently persuaded me that I
could accomplish more than I am capable of.

—Chip Caldwell

To the patients God has entrusted us to serve.

—Charles Denham, M.D.

Table of Contents

Acknowledgments

First and foremost, we wish to acknowledge the breakthrough work of Don Berwick, M.D., president of the Institute for Healthcare Improvement. From the beginning of the quality movement in healthcare in the late 1980s and continuing with his work with the Institute of Medicine (IOM), he has shown leadership in innovating solutions in the detection, mitigation, and prevention of adverse events and medical errors.

Second, we wish to express our appreciation to those at Premier who aided our work. CEO Richard Norling, by making patient safety a critical priority, chartering a senior leadership team to gather data and craft solutions, and establishing a strategic partnership with the Institute for Healthcare Improvement, paved the way for rapid knowledge discovery. Joan Crouze and Joyce White at the Resource Center in Charlotte, North Carolina, were instrumental in keeping us up to date on the most recent discussions and articles on medication errors, which became an almost insurmountable task after the release of the IOM report, *To Err Is Human.* Jim Scott and Herb Kuhn provided constant analyses of news articles and the reaction in Washington and also organized critical visits with Senator Frist and his staff and the Agency for Healthcare Research and Quality. Don Kendzierski, Ross Edwards, and Bert Patterson provided much-needed leadership in the medication error reduction collaborative among hospitals. Greg Archer constructed and analyzed web-based best practice data collection, and Carolyn Harris provided much-needed organization of interviews, material collection, and survey analysis production.

Many healthcare leaders eagerly shared their time, ideas, and reactions in the preparation of this manuscript. These include, among others, Barbara Spreadbury of SSM; Jim Reinertsen, M.D., CEO of CareGroup, in Boston; Keith Martin, M.D., chief medical officer of Legacy Health System in Portland, Oregon; Victor Perini of Methodist Health System in Memphis, Tennessee; Jeanne Ezelli of Blount Memorial Hospital in Maryville, Tennessee; the staff at Bridge Medical in San Diego, California; and Sherry Anderson, R.N., at St. Mary's Medical Center in Madison, Wisconsin.

Tom Nolan and Jim Espinoza, M.D., continue to contribute idealized design, change concept construction, and culture and belief system analysis in the quest for error reduction techniques.

The staff at Health Care Concepts in Austin, Texas—particularly, Kevin Cook, Frank Guilloteau, Rod Reyna and John Latino—provided critical research, analysis, and editing work.

We also wish to thank the staff at Health Administration Press, in particular Audrey Kaufman, Cami Cacciatore, Robert Fromberg, and Renee Anderson, who not only provided much-needed editorial and architectural guidance but also kept us moving forward to get the manuscript to press.

Preface

ALMOST NO ONE associated with the healthcare industry for any period of time, particularly those of us who have suffered through medical or administrative call rotations, was truly surprised by the report on medical errors published by the Institute of Medicine (IOM) in *To Err Is Human* (Kohn, Corrigan, and Donaldson 1999). Even the IOM's projected death rate from adverse events of up to 98,000 deaths per year—the equivalent of one Boeing 747 crash every 16 hours—was not questioned because we all know the healthcare industry is fraught with complexity, is often chaotic, and has significant system design flaws.

And although defect management might not be given as much priority in the healthcare industry as it is in other industries, most healthcare professionals believe that much progress has been made. For example, the Institute for Safe Medication Practices, the Massachusetts Hospital Association, the Healthcare Advisory Board, the Institute for Healthcare Improvement, and the Veterans Administration, to name only a few, have been providing analysis, solutions databases, and dialoging forums for more than four years. Moreover, the U.S. Pharmacopeia Medication Errors Reporting Program has been in existence for more than ten years. Perhaps the real value of the IOM report is that it has elevated the issue to its proper strategic perspective on the senior leadership agenda, bringing the issue of adverse events and medical errors into executive suites and boardrooms across America.

When planning this book, we debated among ourselves, with our publishers, and with those who helped provide recommended solutions, whether to include all categories of adverse events and medical errors or, instead, to focus on the more limited area of adverse drug events and medication errors. In the end, we decided a focus on adverse drug events and medication error reduction is more appropriate at this time because there is widespread agreement on possible solutions.

The problems, and the reasons we undertook this work, were many, at least based on our observations and discussions with CEOS and other senior leaders in the healthcare industry. First, although the healthcare industry maintains numerous databases for the detection, prevention, and mitigation of adverse drug events and medication errors, it seems to lack a quality-based methodology to approach the issue. We believe a unifying methodology is needed to clarify organizational aims, establish databases of process interventions to attack errors, provide tools and techniques to execute these interventions, and, finally, to track whether gains are made and maintained.

Second, most CEOS and senior leaders seem to lack an appreciation for the cost recovery potential offered by an error reduction strategy. In one interview, for example, the leader of a major health system reporting significant progress in reducing medication errors admitted that, although in retrospect the cost of the errors was obvious, the system leaders had not only failed to consider the cost recovery potential but also believed that the recovery of those costs would have been impossible without substantial additional data collection and process redesign.

The quality revolution in the manufacturing industry, of course, was embedded in the concept that "as quality goes up, costs go down." The cost of defects, warranties, and lost customers has been a mainstay strategy that has evolved into the current wave of Six Sigma Quality programs at leading U.S. companies such as GE, Motorola, Mercury Motors, and SeaRay. Having capitalized on the industrial quality movement spurred by the Japanese in the '80s and '90s to improve profits through cost reduction initiatives that focused on error and defect reduction, these companies have raised their sights from their current performance at 3 sigma (approximately 66 thousand errors per million occurrences) to attempt near perfection—6 sigma quality (3.4 errors per million occurrences). These pioneers have documented that at 3 sigma defect levels the cost of quality averages between 25 and 30 percent of operating expenses, but drops below 5 percent at 6 sigma levels.

Healthcare process errors, defects, and adverse events also account for significant costs in the form of lost productivity, rework, and inspection of nurses, physicians, and others involved in direct patient care, not to mention costs resulting from malpractice issues and cost avoidance measures.

Of course, these costs are above and beyond those associated with alleviating and managing the loss of public, community, and patient confidence in the healthcare system and the effect of human suffering. Therefore, we felt it essential to explore strategies not only to reduce adverse drug events and medication errors, but to also ensure cost recovery.

However, a disclaimer is in order. The evolution of a system of care that is safe from defect, of high quality, and optimally efficient is currently outside the vision of most healthcare providers and architects. Despite bold talk about progress, much remains to be done and time is of the essence. We offer this book now because we feel a great urgency to find workable solution sets in the public domain to address the needs discussed here.

Finally, although we consider our work viable, we do not offer it or our recommendations as being anything close to a final solution. Indeed, we consider the work evolutionary and in need of constant innovation. Offered in this spirit, we are proud of our recommended approaches but remain humbled by the magnitude of the effort that will be required by all of us.

—*Chip Caldwell and Charles Denham*, M.D.

REFERENCE

Kohn, L.T., J.M. Corrigan, and M.S. Donaldson (eds.). 1999. *To Err Is Human: Building a Safer Health System*. Washington, D.C.: National Academy Press.

Foreword

THE COVER FOR this book should include the admonition: "Warning! Reading this book could change your life!" Let us hope it does. The perilous state of safety in healthcare is both tragic and indefensible; repair is urgently needed. If they were still skeptical, healthcare executives who read this book will no longer be able to escape the conclusion that they have a very major challenge to deal with. Nothing short of total reengineering will do the job. Chip Caldwell and Charles Denham offer guidance as to how to accept that challenge.

The magnitude of the problem of patient safety came to public attention suddenly and dramatically in November, 1999 with the release of the Institute of Medicine (IOM) report, *To Err Is Human*. No report from the IOM, or, for that matter, from any organization, has provoked a comparable public response. Some have said that it is for this century what the Flexner report was for the last. While that might be the hyperbole of zealots, the impact of the report was impressive, and most would agree that making healthcare safe is as important as educating doctors. Policymakers were galvanized. Congress appropriated $50 million to establish a Center for Patient Safety within the Agency for Health Research and Quality.

The IOM urged hospitals and healthcare systems to make error prevention a priority, to establish safety programs, and to implement known best practices for safety. It emphasized the importance of active involvement by the leadership of organizations to create the new nonpunitive culture of safety and to redesign systems. The report reemphasized what every safe industry has learned—that human errors are not caused by lax and careless people, but are the end result of multiple complex and inter-connected system failures. All of our systems are at fault: training and education; design of processes, equipment, and facilities; management, working conditions; and the way professionals and personnel interact.

But healthcare has an additional burden. Sanctified by tradition and decades of practice, doctors and nurses have not only placed all of the responsibility for safety on individual practitioners rather than on the design of systems, but have reinforced that responsibility with shame and punishment. Instead of a culture of safety, the culture of blame creates an atmosphere of fear and self-reproach that leads nurses and doctors to hide mistakes and be dishonest with their patients and themselves. Because we do not talk about our mistakes, we do not learn from them and are therefore doomed to repeat them. Changing this culture is the greatest challenge of all.

How does one change a culture? How does one reengineer the systems? Clearly, change is a management responsibility. Doctors and nurses alone cannot change the systems they work within. They must be an integral part of the redesign of those systems and implementation of changes—but they need direction, support, and resources. Safety has to become a priority for management. The organization must become a learning organization, and both managers and employees need to learn to think in systems terms. Safety has to become everyone's responsibility. Chip Caldwell and Charles Denham have some ideas about how to do that, and have focused on medication safety as an example of the type of systems reengineering that needs to be done.

While this book is packed with many ideas and concepts, two that are particularly useful may be new to many readers. The first is the observation that there is no clear one-to-one relationship between medication errors and injuries. Traditionally, nurses have stressed the "Five Rights"—the right drug, dose, route, time, patient—but many injuries, which we call adverse drug events, result from other causes, or at the least are not fully under the nurse's control. A major share of adverse drug events, for example, are due to prescribing errors. Conversely, the vast majority of medication errors (perhaps 95 percent or more) do not result in patient harm. Attention to the information management systems and developing methods that do not depend solely on human vigilance have been found to be much more efficacious than further training or rigid control of nursing practices. Changing the industry's way of thinking is a major challenge.

The second concept that many readers will find especially useful is "recapturing lost productivity." While no one questions our responsibility to do everything we can to reduce the risk of injury to our patients, in such a fiercely competitive environment many worry about finding the resources.

Fear no more. Savings abound, and Caldwell and Denham show you how to capture them. They demonstrate how reducing adverse events by systems redesign increases productivity, and then they show the reader how to take the next step that is so often ignored: matching staffing to reduced demand. The result is that value, the quotient of quality over costs, increases as quality rises and costs fall. The vision is clear: we can be safe and save money at the same time. It is not easy, but it is doable.

Most of all this is an action manual. The core is the "100-Day Plan" in which the principles and practices are brought to action under the framework of clearly defined objectives in a specified program to achieve the aims. The last chapter provides tools for self-assessment and planning based on the concepts and lessons presented earlier. All of the chapters are packed with valuable material that will benefit from repeated readings and reference.

It is an exciting time for those concerned with making healthcare safe—which is every one of us! At last there is a national concern, the beginning of commitment of resources, and awareness among healthcare professionals and managers that we can do better. We know much about what we can do to make healthcare safer. Improved practices are being developed and disseminated rapidly. We owe it to our patients and to ourselves to embrace these new methods and to change from a culture of blame to a culture of safety.

—*Lucian L. Leape, M.D.*
Harvard School of Public Health

CHAPTER ONE

Introduction

The team that makes the fewest mistakes wins.

—Chan Caldwell, Assistant Football Coach,
University of Tennessee, 1951

M EDICATION SAFETY AND COST RECOVERY advocates a defined management methodology known as the 100-Day Plan, a four-step approach to achieving a dramatic improvement in current integrated delivery network (IDN) and medical center performance. Early successes at a number of organizations leading the effort and considerable research into the quality successes of other industries such as the American automobile industry that have faced and overcome similar quality problems, demonstrate that the challenge can be broken down into three critical components:

1. Transforming the organization's belief system, as observed by Don Berwick, M.D., president of the Institute for Healthcare Improvement (IHI), from one that accepts that "errors are a part of medicine" and surrenders to poor quality to one that declares war on errors, even to six sigma levels (3.4 errors per million opportunity for error);
2. Dedicating adequate resources to knowledge management (including executive commitment, mitigating technology, training, and strategic redirection) to produce and implement a constantly improving adverse drug event and medication error change concepts database; and
3. Recapturing the productivity lost and cost surrendered because of high error rates, estimated by many in the industry to be as high as 40 percent of the healthcare organization's operating expenses (Harry and Schroeder 1999).

This book is intended for the healthcare management team: those individuals charged with reducing adverse drug events and medication errors; the chief financial officer (CFO) and those charged with balancing the effects of declining reimbursement; and others passionate about the improvement of quality, the reduction of errors, and the recapture of lost productivity and cost.

MANDATE TO FIND SOLUTIONS

The reasons why adverse drug events and medication errors have become an accepted complexity of physician practice have been postulated over the past several months since the Institute of Medicine (IOM) report on medical errors made its way into American medical circles, community hospital boardrooms, IDN executive management sessions, and even local newspapers. Some theorists suggest that medical error is an unavoidable byproduct of care because medical care is so complex, patient conditions are so individual, and life in acute care settings is so spontaneous and unpredictable. Others suggest that because physicians practice independently, no single physician experiences a disturbing rate of error and thus no alarm system exists for the profession as a whole.

The reasons why adverse drug events and medication errors have become an accepted complexity of nursing and pharmacy practice are being explored as well. Some suggest that nurses and pharmacists are directed to orient care toward physicians and, historically, have been discouraged from being aggressive about questioning orders. In fact, in several recent incidents, nursing and pharmacy personnel questions about therapeutic regimens were overridden by physician orders. Others suggest that errors are dramatically underreported because caregivers have been made to feel personally ashamed if an error occurs on their watch.

Also a mystery are the reasons why healthcare CEOs, governing board members, and executives have failed to engage quality and error reduction to drive productivity gain during times of aggressive cost reduction, as did their peers in the automobile and manufacturing industries in the 1980s and 1990s. Some suggest that healthcare executives, even physician CEOs, are too far removed from direct-care practices to experience the quality, safety, and productivity relationships that executives in other industries experience. Others suggest that the misalignment of reimbursement paradigms in the healthcare industry produces different success factors for all constituents—physicians, HMOs, employers, and health system leaders alike—that prevent a vantage point from which errors become visible, critical, and manageable. In other industries, warranty costs, costs of poor quality and defects, and production costs all come together on the CEO's desk.

In healthcare, reimbursement practices across the continuum of care are often in conflict and are not managed by one single CEO.

However, the world has changed. The blinders have been removed and the problem is widely known by our most vital customer: the patient. And through the media, political agendas, and special-interest and business action groups, our customers have aggregated to drive for solutions.

EFFECTS OF ADVERSE DRUG EVENTS AND MEDICATION ERRORS

Although it is perhaps obvious, it is important to note that adverse drug events, the most significant subset of medication errors, should receive the lion's share of the change effort. Adverse drug events and other types of adverse events, by definition, can harm patients, sometimes catastrophically. Thus, adverse drug events drive most of the cost of poor quality and lost productivity. Medication errors other than adverse drug events should not be ignored, however. As revealed in subsequent chapters of this book, medication errors, by definition, do not harm patients and do not consume as many precious healthcare resources as adverse drug events do. Nonetheless, they are a hidden drain on resources, negatively affecting staff morale and causing patient unrest. Unlike other categories of errors, medication errors have been the object of reduction work for many years. In fact, a uniformly acknowledged change concepts database enjoys wide circulation among many leading researchers and organizations. The database of sentinel events maintained by the Joint Commission on Accreditation of Healthcare Organizations ranks medication errors at 11 percent, second only to inpatient suicide (Goldfield and Nash 1999). The incidence of adverse drug events has been reported to be as low as 1.8 percent, but the broader issue of total medication errors has been reported to be as high as 20 percent when multiple detection methods of self-reporting, automated systems, and manual audits are combined to discover occurrence levels (Clinical Initiatives Center 1999).

A variety of factors account for the prevalence of underreporting in the industry, including:

- a fear of reporting;
- a reluctance to use the burdensome, time-consuming reporting procedures; and
- the shame of admitting that an error has occurred.

According to a Clinical Initiatives Center survey in 1999, 38 percent of medication errors were never reported to senior management and 23

Lost airline bag

ADE

	Lost work injury per workweek			Airline near-miss collisions
Error Rate	1/100	1/1000	1/10,000	1/M
Sigma Level	3σ	4σ	5σ	6σ

percent of adverse events were not filed with the organizations' incident-reporting system (Clinical Initiatives Center 1999).

Moreover, we have some idea of the cost of poor quality resulting from adverse drug events and medication errors. The Clinical Initiatives Center study also revealed that patients who experience an adverse drug event stay in the hospital for 23.9 days, compared to 8.8 days for patients who do not experience an adverse event. Another study at a 400-bed institution with 15,500 admissions estimated that adverse events and complications consumed $16.4 million, or about 2.5 percent of the institution's operating budget. Adverse drug events, anesthesia accidents, and surgical errors combined to produce 65 percent of the total cost of all adverse events (Clinical Initiatives Center 1999).

The rate of errors, defects, and adverse events in healthcare compared to other industries is remarkable, so much so that other industries would be unable to survive if their rates approximated those in healthcare. This was demonstrated recently by Tom Nolan (2000a), a leading thinker in reliability engineering (see Figure 1.1).

The added cost attributable to errors would price their goods and services beyond the consumers' means. In every other industry, error rates are among the key indicators tracked by the CEO. Yet, in healthcare, except for a few notable exceptions, CEOs are provided no such data.

Figure 1.2 further illustrates the locus of errors by subprocess, percentage intercepted, and potential for cost recovery as a result of medication error reduction.

FIGURE 1.2.   MEDICAL ERROR ANALYSIS

	Physician Prescribing	Order Processing	Drug Preparation	Drug Administration	Drug Monitoring
Error Occurrence Percent	39 %	12 %	11 %	38 %	NA
Percent Error Interrupted	48 %	33 %	34 %	2 %	NA
Potential Productivity Recapture	High	Medium	Low	High	High

THE ATTACK ON ERROR REDUCTION

Tom Nolan and Don Berwick suggest that the attack on error reduction encompass three elements (Nolan 2000b):

1. preventing errors before they occur;
2. making errors visible so they can be detected; and
3. mitigating the effects of errors that are not prevented.

To realize our aim, Nolan further indicates that the design of safe systems enables us to engage five tactics that:

1. reduce complexity;
2. optimize information processing;
3. automate wisely;
4. use constraints; and
5. mitigate the unwanted side effects of change.

Research for this book involved interviews with leaders from many healthcare organizations that have successfully reduced adverse drug events and medication errors and have used proven methodologies to solve generic quality issues. Those organizations that are recognized as the safest, highest-quality, and most cost-effective healthcare institutions share the following characteristics:

- They set and achieve "stretch" goals that, at the outset, appear to be unachievable. Successful institutions share a belief in the impossible.
- They approach problems with a sense of urgency. As IHI expressed it, "What can you do by next Tuesday?" (Nolan and Haraden 2000).
- They do not view status quo as an option (Leape et al. 1998). As Tom Peters (1982) discovered during his interviews with the leaders of America's most successful companies for *In Search of Excellence* more than a decade ago, successful institutions have "a bias for action."
- They encourage senior management to exhibit a "firm intention to succeed" (Berwick 2000).
- They have mastered a disciplined methodology, such as the 100-Day Plan management method.
- They post monthly measures that document the linkage between activity and results.
- Finally, they are dedicated to continuously enhancing the medication error reduction change concepts database.

CONTENT

This book touches on the most pressing measures required to dramatically reduce medication errors and adverse drug events and to recapture the costs associated with them. Chapter 2 "Magnitude of the Problem" addresses the current state of knowledge regarding the nature of error. Chapter 3 "Accelerators and Inhibitors" considers accelerating and inhibiting factors in the institution's quest to reduce adverse drug events and medication errors. Chapter 4 "The 100-Day Plan" explains the 100-Day Plan management method, including the infrastructure it requires, measurement approaches, idealized design implementation steps, knowledge management, and how to hold gains. Chapter 5 "Knowledge Management Loop for Medication Error Reduction" discusses the theory of medication error change concepts and the current thinking of leading organizations. Chapter 6 "Knowledge Management Loop to Match Staffing to Demand" describes techniques that healthcare institutions can use to recapture lost productivity. Chapter 7 "Closing the Gaps" contains self-assessments and planning guides to strengthen existing approaches.

In summary, as the public mandates, the healthcare industry, like other industries, must aggressively attack medication errors and adverse drug events to recapture the productivity costs incurred by these errors in the process.

REFERENCES

Berwick, D. *Personal interview.* November 18, 2000.

Clinical Initiatives Center. 1999. *Prescription for Change: Toward a Higher Standard in Medication Management.* Washington, DC: The Advisory Board Company.

Goldfield, N., and D. Nash (eds.). 1999. *Managing Quality of Care in a Cost-focused Environment.* Tampa, FL: American College of Physician Executives.

Harry, M., and R. Schroeder. 1999. *Six Sigma, The Breakthrough Management Strategy Revolutionizing the World's Top Corporations.* New York: Doubleday.

Leape, L., A. Kabcenell, D. Berwick, and J. Roessner. 1998. *Reducing Adverse Events.* Boston: Institute for Healthcare Improvement.

Nolan, T. 2000a. "Design of Safe Systems." Paper presented at the Premier–Institute for Healthcare Improvement Medication Management Idealized Design Conference, Boston, April 27–28.

———. 2000b. "System Changes to Improve Patient Safety." *British Medical Journal* 320: 771–73.

Nolan, T., and C. Haraden. 2000. "Idealized Design of the Medication Management System." Paper presented at the Premier–Institute for Healthcare Improvement Medication Management Idealized Design Conference, Boston, April 27–28.

Peters, J., and R. H. Waterman, Jr. 1982. *In Search of Excellence: Lessons From America's Best-run Companies.* New York: Warner Books.

CHAPTER TWO

Magnitude of the Problem

The important thing is not to stop questioning.

—Albert Einstein

T HIS CHAPTER EXAMINES the current state of knowledge regarding the nature, sources, and underlying causes of medication errors and adverse drug events and provides some examples of error prevention practices that have been applied successfully in the aviation industry. The aim is to provide leaders in the healthcare industry with information they can use to implement a management system dedicated to systematically reducing medication errors and adverse drug events.

When patients enter healthcare facilities, they expect to receive responsive, high-quality, safe, and appropriate care. Trust is the most important element of the provider-patient relationship. Until recently, the last thing on most patients' minds has been the possibility of being the victims of preventable harm during the course of care delivery.

THREE CRITICAL ISSUES

The reality is that preventable adverse drug events are indeed a major issue in healthcare. There are three critical "A's" to addressing the challenge:

- *Awareness.* Suppliers, providers, and purchasers of healthcare must become aware of the magnitude, systemic nature, and real consequences of adverse events. They must understand that there is very little overlap between what we traditionally think of as medication errors and the adverse drug events that cause harm to patients.

- *Accountability.* Without focused, personal accountability on the part of administrative and medical leaders and their commitment to make patient safety a major strategic imperative, little sustained improvement is possible. Healthcare has become very complex and is fraught with distributed and diluted accountability.
- *Action.* Patient safety initiatives are difficult to launch. Few off-the-shelf solutions and even fewer technologies can be employed without a systems approach. As is discussed in this chapter, any action or innovation should be founded on three critical elements:
  -It must be grounded in a safety culture.
  -It must reengineer care and operational processes.
  -It must apply human factors science.

Clearly, patients and other healthcare stakeholders are unaware of the potential for unnecessary harm and suffering caused by iatrogenic injuries (injuries induced inadvertently by a physician or surgeon or by medical treatment or diagnostic procedures)—yet the problem is the reality of healthcare today (Runciman and Moller 2000).

MEDICATION ERRORS AND ADVERSE EVENTS

Although definitions vary, a medication error is typically considered to be a mistake in the five "R's": right drug to the right patient at the right time through the right route at the right dose. Unfortunately, the adverse drug events that cause harm and extend hospital stays with a consequence of increased expense are not generally caused by what we traditionally think of as the five "R's." Rather, harm is frequently caused by a lack of information at the time of patient assessment, during transitions between care settings, or because of unrecognized clinical issues that should change a course in therapy.

Research on the Magnitude of the Problem

The misconception concerning the magnitude of the problem had been unappreciated by the public until the media began to publish research on the issue. The Institute of Medicine (IOM) report, *To Err is Human: Building a Safer Health Care System,* published in late 1999, was clearly a turning point (Kohn, Corrigan, and Donaldson 1999).

Two significant studies are often quoted regarding the effect of adverse events—one was conducted in Colorado and Utah hospitals (Thomas 2000), and the other is the Harvard Medical Practice Study (HMPS), which examined hospitals in New York (Brennan et al. 1991). The Utah Colorado study (UTCO) found that 8.8 percent of adverse events led to death, whereas HMPS found that 13.6 percent of adverse events in New York hospitals resulted in fatal outcomes. In both studies, over half of these adverse events resulted from preventable medical errors.

Adverse drug events were found to be the most frequent category of harm following surgical complications in the HMPS and UTCO which reported, respectively, that 0.72 percent and 0.5 percent of admissions suffered adverse drug events.

When extrapolated to the more than 33.6 million admissions to U.S. hospitals in 1997, the results of these studies imply that at least 44,000 Americans die each year as a result of medical errors (Thomas et al. 1999; AHA 1999). The results of the Harvard Medical Practice Study suggest that the number may be as high as 98,000 (Brennan et al. 1991; AHA 1999). Even when using the lower estimate, deaths attributable to medical errors exceed the number attributable to the eighth leading cause of death. More people die in a given year as a result of medical errors than as a result of motor vehicle accidents (43,458), breast cancer (42,297), or AIDS (16,516) (Centers for Disease Control and Prevention 1999).

Critics of the Harvard Medical Practice Study and the subsequent IOM publication have stated that the data overestimate the seriousness of the problem. The Harvard study's most serious limitation is that it is a retrospective medical review, which relies on information extracted from medical records, most likely leading to a substantial underestimation of the prevalence of injury (Leape 2000).

Detractors have criticized the published reports for having a hostile tone. For example, they described the message from IOM as "harsh and shrill" or found that such reports imply that the American healthcare system has lost its status as being "world-class" (McDonald, Weiner, and Hui 2000). A review of the medication errors and adverse event literature indicates higher numbers than found in the HMPS and UTCO studies. Two major studies by Classen et al. (1997) and Bates et al. (1995) reported that 2.43 percent and 6.5 percent of admissions resulted in adverse drug events, respectively. While the variation may be attributable to methodology, definition, and institution-specific issues, these studies still support that the problem is significantly greater than previously believed.

Accountability

The development of the American healthcare system has evolved into a complex and fragmented set of systems suffering from distributed and therefore diluted accountability. We have become more technology based, and criticism of the system is not an indictment of the people within it but, rather, of a system that needs to address performance improvement with a systems approach using technology as an enabler.

Some feel that certain reports do not validate the ongoing medication error research and quality improvement (QI) initiatives that have occurred during the past four decades. In the early 1960s, researchers began conducting comprehensive medication error studies and publishing the results in professional journals. Hospital risk managers, pharmacy and therapeutic committees, and QI teams have worked diligently to address these concerns, often with few resources other than their own time and energy.

The second IOM report, *Crossing the Quality Chasm* (2001a), maintains that there is still much work to be done to improve the quality of the U.S. healthcare system and that safety problems are just the "tip of the iceberg." The report suggests that a redesign of the healthcare system be based on three principles and six aims. The principles include the requirements that the redesign effort apply evidence-based medicine, be patient-centered in focus, and take a systems approach. The report outlines six major aims for healthcare reform, the first of which is patient safety. The other five aims are effectiveness, patient-centeredness, timeliness, efficiency, and equity.

Dr. Bill Runciman, leader of the Australian Patient Safety Foundation, is an intensive care specialist and an international leader in the patient safety movement. He frequently compares the risk of participating as a patient in the healthcare system with that of participating in perceived high-risk activities. In his keynote address "Building Systems That Do No Harm: Advancing Patient Safety Through Partnership and Share Knowledge" at the National Patient Safety Symposium held in Dallas, Texas, in June 2000, Runciman noted that the risk of death (per 100 million hours' exposure) from being a patient in an Australian hospital is 20 times greater than the risk of death from flying in a commercial aircraft. Using the same metric, the risk of death from elective abdominal surgery is ten times greater than the risk of death from skydiving, and the same risk from emergency abdominal surgery is one hundred times greater than the risk of death from skydiving. The reality presented by these statistics is that hospitals can be complex and dangerous places.

The bottom line is that adverse events from medical errors, and specifically medication errors, are relatively uncommon and diffused over the millions of care processes that occur in our care facilities. However, they are very common when compared to the incidence of the diseases we treat. Medical adverse events leading to harm are a significant and critical problem that must command as much attention as any major disease. At the end of the day, our moral contract with our patients is that we "do no harm."

Business Case

For the less altruistic caregivers, the language of economics may be more effective than an appeal to noble sensibilities. The question then should be: Is there a business case for safety and adverse event reduction? The answer is an emphatic and absolute yes!

Total national costs (lost income, lost household production, disability, and healthcare costs) of preventable adverse events are estimated to be between $17 billion and $29 billion, of which direct healthcare costs represent over one-half (Thomas et al. 1999). In terms of lives lost, patient safety is as important an issue as worker safety. Every year, more than 6,000 Americans die from workplace injuries (OSHA 1998). Adverse drug events alone, occurring in or out of the hospital, are estimated to account for more than 7,000 deaths annually (Phillips, Christenfeld, and Glynn 1998).

According to the Harvard Medical Practice Study, nearly 4 percent of patients suffered an injury that either prolonged their hospital stay or resulted in disability, and nearly 14 percent of the injuries were fatal (Leape et al. 1991b). Extrapolating these results to the entire United States would attribute 180,000 deaths each year to iatrogenic injuries. Further investigations into these injuries revealed that 53 percent of these errors were preventable (Leape et al. 1991).

With the advent of reimbursement mechanisms such as per diem methods, many downstream costs generated by adverse events are shifted to hospitals. There are many discharge categories where an adverse event can convert a "margin-positive case" to a "margin-negative case." Clearly, there is a substantial business case for reducing errors on the expense side.

How about the revenue side? As safety becomes a differentiator to the best-informed consumers, hospitals with legitimate safety programs will be rewarded with their patronage. With the advent of the Internet and the intense focus of 24-hour news media, there is an increasing power of patient choice fueled by information. Some of the information is of high quality, but much of it is not. A legitimate patient safety program is of tremendous real value, even if solely as a driver of successful marketing campaigns. In the future, access to standardized healthcare quality indicators at regional and national levels will have a direct effect on patient choice.

The third and most recent IOM report, *Envisioning the National Health Care Quality Report* (2001b), provides insight into the measures that will be used to gauge the quality of our healthcare system. Healthcare must be safe, effective, patient-centered, and timely. It emphasizes the need for proper quality measures, not just from the policy perspective, but also from the patient's perspective. These measures should reflect the changing needs of the patient/consumer and the impact of the healthcare system across four major areas: prevention, acute care, chronic care, and end-of-life care.

The report will likely be available in several versions, each tailored to a specific group of healthcare stakeholders including providers, purchasers, researchers, policy makers, and patients/consumers. Additionally, it will provide the "quality status" of both the national and regional healthcare systems (Institute of Medicine 2001b).

Finally, the Joint Commission on Accreditation of Healthcare Organizations (JCAHO), which has the responsibility of accrediting hospitals for Medicare reimbursement, has instituted a set of new and revised safety and error reductions standards to be implemented by July 2001 (JCAHO 2000). For example, physicians now must inform patients and their families about the possibility of adverse events. This new focus on patient safety reflects growing recognition and support of the themes delivered in the IOM reports. Being proactive will be key for providers to stay in business.

Effect of Consumerism

Online consumerism is increasingly being recognized as a significant trend in all industries. Generally, informed consumers are more likely to have health insurance. Online consumers are likely to be the segment that helps pay for the healthcare delivered to the indigent. In essence, the old adage of "no margin ... no mission" will never be more true. If your hospital does not attract the people who help pay for charity cases, the harsh reality of red ink brought on by the Balanced Budget Act of 1997 will only be more profound.

Yes, there is a terrific business case for reducing adverse events. And yes, you need to be able to make your business case as strong as possible, no matter how altruistic your institution may be. You need to be able to marshal the greatest investment that you can. Successful safety programs require care process reengineering, education, and enabling technologies. Such comprehensive programs, although not inexpensive, will indeed pay for themselves.

Medication Errors and Adverse Drug Events: Minimal Overlap?

We should make an important distinction between adverse drug events and medication errors. Logic would have us believe that if we were to reduce medication errors in an institution, we would be reducing adverse drug events in patients. However, the limited literature on the subject questions this assumption (Classen 1998). Medication errors, following the strict definition of the "five Rights" (also known as the five "R's"), share little overlap with adverse drug events. A study conducted by Classen et al. (1997) at

LDS Hospital in Salt Lake City, Utah found that less than 1 percent of adverse drug events result from medication errors. A follow-up review based on daily surveillance of 202,222 hospitalized patients identified a 3.5 percent overlap in events classified as both medication errors and adverse drug events (Classen 1999).

Much of the confusion regarding the overlap between medication errors and adverse drug events centers on the definitions applied to each of these terms. If we define an adverse drug event as actual harm to patients and a medication error as making a mistake on the five "R's"—right dose, right patient, right route, right time, and right drug—the issue crystallizes. The medical literature indicates that most medication errors do not result in harm to patients and most harm to patients is not the result of a failure to get one of the five "R's" correct.

This can have a dramatic effect on the published incidences of the errors and events. Using a broader definition which includes patient assessment and ordering errors, Bates et al. (1995) found 530 medication errors in 379 admissions—or 1.4 medication error per admission, and a 19 percent overlap between adverse drug events and errors. Classen, in his follow up, found only 4,155 medication errors for 202,222 per patient, or less than 2 percent.

The confusion between medication errors and adverse drug events can hinder efforts to reduce adverse drug events (Classen 1999). Although medication errors have garnered the bulk of media and public attention, it is adverse drug events that cause actual harm to patients. One study has shown that substantial reductions in adverse drug events can be attained through the use of computerized surveillance systems that provide rapid feedback to clinicians, track drug allergies, and automatically calculate important physiological parameters such as renal clearance. It demonstrated a 70 percent reduction in antibiotic-related adverse drug events when such an automatic surveillance system was used in the hospital setting (Evans et al. 1998).

Furthermore, there is a noteworthy study by Bates et al. (1998) that evaluated systems to mitigate serious medication errors. It showed that reduction of medication errors impacted potential adverse drug events by 84 percent but was not statistically conclusive in reducing preventable adverse drug events. Because of the dearth of evidence in this area and varying definitions, it would be premature to discount medication error prevention strategies as ineffective in addressing the adverse drug event problem.

Most adverse drug events are the result of some type of information failure, such as inaccurate dosing, failure to recognize potentially harmful interactions, and other informatics failures. However, these failures have little to do with the logistical issues surrounding the five "R's." Therefore, if we strive to perfect how information is gathered, processed, and handled throughout the medication process, rather than perfecting the five "R's", we will be addressing the cause of most of the harm patients suffer because of adverse drug events.

Not all drug-related problems harm patients, but those that do are costly. Drug-related morbidity and mortality has been estimated to cost the United States from $30.1 billion to $136 billion a year (Johnson and Bootman 1995). According to the Physician Insurers Association of America, the average indemnity payment for a medical malpractice claim related to medication errors is $99,721 (1993). Other studies have suggested that preventable adverse drug events prolong length of stay (LOS) an average of 4.6 days (Bates et al. 1997); add more than $2,000 to $4,600 to the cost of hospitalization; and almost triple the risk of death even after adjustment for severity of illness (Kohn, Corrigan, and Donaldson 1999; Classen et al. 1997; Flynn and Barker 2000). For a large medical center, this amounts to a cost of between $1.5 million and $3.9 million annually. Extrapolated to the entire country, medication-related problems have the potential to cost as much $2 billion per year (Kohn, Corrigan, and Donaldson 1999).

Although adverse drug events result in a significant number of deaths and injuries, there is a considerable lack of concern and understanding of how to prevent them. This lack of awareness is because adverse drug events initially appear to be isolated events. The reports of poor clinical outcomes because of adverse drug events are often perceived as anecdotal situations rather than indications of serious systemic problems. Moreover, the lack of response in the past from both government support systems and medical associations has not served to prioritize the problem. The tendency within the medical profession to protect its own has made medical societies and hospitals reluctant to make errors known to the public or to take actions against those involved (Helmreich and Merrit 1998).

Causes of Adverse Drug Events and Medication Errors

The causes of adverse drug events and medication errors are many and complex. A review of the medical literature available on this topic can be both confusing and frustrating.

At the time of preparing this manuscript, one of the authors, Charles R. Denham, M.D., CEO of Health Care Concepts, Inc. (HCC) was participating in an extensive review of the entire area. Recognizing a tremendous opportunity for quality improvement for its more than 1,800 hospitals, Richard Norling, CEO of Premier, Inc., one of the country's largest group purchasing organizations, established a long-term collaborative relationship with the Institute for Healthcare Improvement (IHI) led by Donald M. Berwick, M.D. This initiative, known as the Medication Management Idealized Design

Project, is under way as a joint initiative between the Premier Innovation Institute team, IHI, and a number of world-class institutions. The initiative is composed of two elements: a discovery effort focused on defining the requirements of world-class performance, and development of an ideal design that could deliver breakthrough performance.

The discovery effort led by HCC uses a "map, gap, plug, and play" cycle approach. The first step is to map an "is state" (current state) of integrated clinical and operational processes. The second step is to undertake an evidence-based medicine approach to identify the gaps, consisting of the "hazard zones" or areas in the system where there is a high concentration of adverse drug events. In the third step, the existing "enabling solutions" (products, services, and technologies) that can reduce adverse drug events will be identified, again using an evidence-based medicine approach to define the performance, and then plugged in as remedies. The final step is to play the full story out to the provider and supplier communities in an effort to engage them in coproducing the enabling solutions that currently do not exist but could prevent or minimize adverse drug events. A rapid process improvement approach is used to continuously repeat the cycle.

The methods used in the discovery effort are the same methods used by Premier to place innovative breakthrough products under contract. Tom Nolan, Ph.D. and Carol Haraden, Ph.D., are providing the leadership on behalf of IHI for the idealized design effort. After the effort has been completed, the goal is to take the learning and provide the concepts, tools, and resources to the Premier Clinical Performance Initiatives targeting 1,800 hospitals and led by Dr. Jack Cox on behalf of Premier.

Workgroups focused on the discovery effort have used the integrated process maps created by IHI through its Breakthrough Series as a starting point. We have added to the maps and have begun to elucidate clear hazard zones. With the assistance of recognized experts such as David C. Classen, M.D., and Lucian L. Leape, M.D., certain patterns are becoming clearer.

Adverse drug events occur more commonly at certain steps along the care process: transitions between care settings such as from the ER, ICU, or OR to nursing units, from outpatient to inpatient settings, or from acute care to extended-care facilities. An adverse drug event study conducted at Luther-Midelfort Hospital in Eau Claire, Wisconsin, also found that 56 percent of the hospital's medication errors occurred at the "interfaces of care," which were identified as the admission process, in-hospital transfers, and at discharge. By focusing on these key areas, the hospital was able to decrease its medication error rate by 82 percent (Rebillot 2000).

Roger Resar, M.D., a physician at the above institution, has received steadfast support by the hospital administration and is pioneering the use of a screening tool for detection of adverse drug events that could empower hospitals to identify process improvement and adverse drug event reduction strategies. The use of this tool has been enhanced and refined through the Premier-IHI Idealized Design Initiative.

A major cause of adverse drug events is the lack of critical information at the time of clinical assessment. Both prior to ordering medication and after a medication has become part of a care plan, the clinical circumstances of the patient have changed and have not been appreciated.

Lesar and his colleagues' review of medication prescribing errors found an overall error rate of 3.9 clinically significant prescribing errors per 1,000 orders over a one-year period. The most common errors found were (Lesar, Briceland, and Stein 1997):

- failure to alter drug therapy in patients with impaired renal or hepatic function (13.9 percent);
- failure to recognize a patient's allergy to the prescribed medication class (12.1 percent);
- use of an incorrect drug name, dosage form, or abbreviation (11.4 percent);
- dosage miscalculation (11.1 percent); and
- use of an unusual or atypical, but critical, dosage frequency (10.8 percent).

Additional studies have shown that lack of drug knowledge and lack of patient information account for 60 percent of proximal causes for medication errors (Leape 2000). Failure to review and complete patient information and to reference drug information while prescribing medications can result in a significant risk for adverse drug events.

With the increase in ambulatory care and shorter LOS, patient self-care is also increasingly contributing to medication errors. Studies have shown that only 36 percent of physicians instruct their patients on proper use of medications (Clinical Initiatives Center 1999). Patient education on medications has become increasingly important because patients may not be able to manage complex drug therapies on their own or recognize the symptoms of an adverse drug event. Patients need information on what each medication is for, how to take it, what it looks like, and how it works (Leape 2000).

Other communication problems while prescribing medications include illegible handwriting, not clarifying drug names, the use of apothecary systems instead of metric systems (such as grains versus grams), the use of nonstandard abbreviations (e.g., U for units), and ambiguous or incomplete orders.

Allergies are the most significant problem related to prescribing anti-biotics, nonsteroid anti-inflammatories, anticonvulsants, and diuretics. In addition, excessive dosing and addiction have been identified as problems associated with prescribing narcotic analgesics and minor tranquilizers (Physician Insurers Association of America 1993).

Other proximal causes associated with medication errors include violations of rules, slips and memory lapses, transcription errors, faulty identity checking, faulty interaction with other services, faulty dose checking, infusion pump and parenteral delivery problems, inadequate monitoring, and drug stocking and delivery problems (Cohen 1999a).

Nursing medication administration errors can occur when doses are not dispensed as packaged or are missing from medication carts, or when dispensing and ordering errors go unchallenged. Nurses usually have multiple priorities that cause interruptions while administering medications. Other sources of errors include illegible or unclear orders, medication administration record (MAR) transcription errors, frequent changes in orders, poor communication among nurses, and nurses floating to units where they are unfamiliar with the medications being used (Wakefield et al. 1998).

A lack of competency by nurses in calculating medications is another significant factor in contributing to medication errors. A study in which nurses were administered a medication calculation test found that 81 percent were unable to calculate medication dosages accurately 90 percent of the time and 40 percent scored less than 70 percent accuracy on the test (Bindler and Bayne 1991).

Of dispensing errors, 88 percent involved giving patients the wrong drug or the wrong dose (Cohen 1999b). Pharmacists rank staff work overload because of downsizing as the most significant cause of dispensing errors (Davis and Cohen 1994). Distractions such as ringing telephones, unnecessary conversations, and poorly designed work areas also contributed to error rates. Proximal causes associated with pharmacy-related errors include faulty drug identity checking, preparation errors, rule violations, drug stocking and delivery problems, faulty dose checking, and faulty interaction with other services (Leape et al. 1995).

Pharmacy-provided unit doses have been found to reduce the incidence of errors; however, cost-cutting strategies have eliminated this tactic in many facilities. Computer-generated labels can cause errors if the information is entered inaccurately. Automated dispensing machines can also result in drug selection and dosing errors because there is no system for verifying accuracy (Institute for Safe Medication Practices 1998, 1999).

Although the determination of whether a process is high risk depends on the setting and services delivered, analyses of medical malpractice claims have found that frequent claims related to medication errors include the transfer of patient care responsibilities between caregivers and facilities and the monitoring of patients during and immediately following high-risk procedures (Ferraco and Spath 1999).

One medication error study found that errors occurred most commonly in physician ordering (39 percent) and nursing administration (38 percent). Correct dosing was the most common type of error, and proximal causes associated with medication errors involved lack of knowledge of both drug and patient information. Many of these errors related to ordering, dosing, and knowledge deficits could be reduced with improved information systems (Leape et al. 1995).

Patient type and severity of illness affect the probability of an adverse event occurring or resulting in an injury or death. Among the factors that contribute to adverse events is the patient's LOS: patients with longer LOS had higher rates of adverse events, with the likelihood increasing about 6 percent for each day of hospitalization. The irony in this is that an adverse reaction results in a longer LOS, which increases the patient's risk of experiencing additional adverse events. The patients most at risk for serious injury from adverse events include those with autoimmune disease or otherwise compromised health, including neonates, chemotherapy patients, the frail elderly, and patients taking five or more medications (Bogner 1994).

Labeling and packaging problems are the second most frequent category of medication errors reported to the U.S. Pharmacopeia Medication Errors Reporting Program (U.S. MERP), and account for 20 percent of all reports (Cousins 1995). Product-related problems that have been associated with adverse events include medications with similar names or identical packaging, medications that are not commonly used or prescribed, and allergic reactions (such as to penicillin) and therapeutic monitoring (e.g., lithium, warfarin, digoxin, and theophylline).

Medical equipment also can contribute to adverse events by either directly causing an incident or contributing to human error that causes it (Bogner 1994). Equipment failure can be the result of inadequate training, insufficient maintenance, and, in some cases, poor design. Equipment displays may be difficult to read, parts may become detached, controls may be poorly located or labeled, alarms may be difficult to distinguish, or the operation of the equipment may be illogical and confusing (Cook, Woods, and Miller 1998). The design of drug devices such as automated intravenous compounders and infusion pumps have provided opportunities for misprogramming rates and miscalculating concentrations. The improper setup of fail-safe clamps and IV lines on this equipment also has contributed to medication errors.

FIGURE 2.1.   SAFETY-MINDED COGNITIVE MODEL

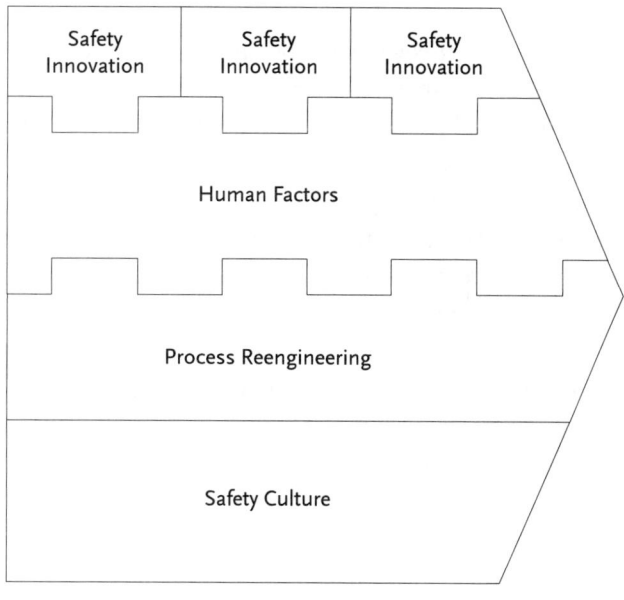

AREAS OF FOCUS

Constructive attention to the reduction of adverse drug events and medication errors through innovative products, services, and technologies requires concentration on distinct, but tightly interrelated, issues that must be grounded in safety. They must be examined in the context of process reengineering, and they must leverage human factors science. These are illustrated in Figure 2.1.

Safety Culture: The Critical Bedrock

Physicians, pharmacists, and nurses are trained to strive for error-free practice. Clinical education focuses on maintaining perfection in both diagnosis and treatment. This need to appear infallible prevents healthcare practitioners from developing the coping skills needed to deal with failures. It inhibits open discussions and analyses of these events. Unlike test pilots, who view errors as inevitable, clinicians view errors as a character fault.

Overlooking mistakes, rather than admitting them, is the only way the facade of perfection can be maintained. The power of denial frequently witnessed in cancer patients is alive and well as a major defense mechanism in our caregivers.

Errors and adverse drug events are usually only discovered when an incident occurs, and the corrective measures that result focus on preventing that particular individual from repeating the same error (Leape 1994). Historically, the measures have been punitive. Hence, a strong feedback loop of blame and shame continually reinforces the behavior.

Physicians typically feel, and not without good reason, that an admission of error leads to censure, increased surveillance, and the appearance of incompetence and carelessness. Intersections of subcultures within medicine, such as between surgeons and anesthesiologists, and breakdowns in team processes also have been identified as problems that contribute to errors (Helmreich and Merrit 1998). Lack of communication among team members, including failure to brief others on the plan for operation, has been identified as yet another common problem that contributes to errors. Other weaknesses in teamwork include lack of leadership and lack of communication regarding alternative courses of action. Often team members are unwilling to inform others of work overload or patient problems and remain silent rather than risk conflict. Moreover, conflicts that occur are not always resolved constructively. Indeed, senior team members do not instruct and mentor less experienced team members as often as might be expected.

Numerous safety champions, such as Leape, have prioritized culture. The lack of emphasis on culture in this chapter is more a reflection of the authors' lack of expertise in the area than of the importance of the issue. Culture and leadership are absolutely critical to addressing performance solutions.

Process Reengineering

The medical approach to error remains based on the concept that properly trained and motivated clinicians do not make errors (OSHA 1998). If clinicians do make errors, the response is equally unforgiving and reactionary: Individuals are found to blame, and tighter controls on their performance are set through an elaborate check system. Errors are perceived as being the result of an individual's lack of sufficient attention or, worse, carelessness (Leape 2000). More training is seen as the solution to the problem, to increase knowledge or introduce more protocols. Another solution is to threaten punishment through reprimands, job termination, or peer disapproval. The civil law system provides punishment for negligence and failure to meet the standard of care. Medical malpractice litigation seeking to tap "deep pockets" drives the argument that the blame lies with whomever has the most assets. Complaints to the state board of medical or nursing examiners also may result in reprimands or licenses being revoked.

Clearly, the delivery of healthcare is a very complex set of interdependent systems with incredibly interlinked and interdependent processes—care process, operational process, and the impact of human fallibility intersect at the point of care. As stated in the second IOM report, *Crossing the Quality Chasm* (2001), improving quality in healthcare can only be achieved by taking a system's approach. It is only by mapping the clinical and operational processes and carefully examining the cause of adverse drug events that significant changes can be made.

Unfortunately, we have a bad case of "magical thinking" regarding high technology products and their ability to provide the quick fix to certain, very complex systems problems. Products, services, technologies, and methods must merely be considered "enabling solutions" that will be secondary to, and enabling of, process reengineering. Reengineering is a systems approach that engages enabling solutions within the context of the underlying systems and processes of care already in place within the organization.

Event Reporting

Event reporting has been the primary means through which adverse drug events have been identified. JCAHO established a Sentinel Event Policy in 1996, in which a sentinel event is defined as one that has resulted in an unanticipated death or major permanent loss of function, not related to the patient's illness or underlying condition (Kohn, Corrigan, and Donaldson 1999). Recently published leadership standards require each accredited organization to define *sentinel event* for its own purpose in establishing mechanisms to identify, report, and manage such events (JCAHO 2000). The most recent JCAHO standards have explicit language about implementing a patient-centered safety program and developing internal programs to educate caregivers (JCAHO 2000). Medication errors have been the most prevalent type of event reported to JCAHO, but a significant barrier to meeting these requirements is insufficient staff participation.

The medication administration standard of the five "R's" is often used to categorize adverse drug event reporting. This system for incident reporting does not reveal the majority of adverse drug events and does not address the underlying causes. Rather, it focuses on the individual associated with the error. The question of who was involved is of less consequence than what went wrong, how, and why (Cohen 1999a). All hospital medication error incident reporting, whether voluntary or mandatory, has suffered from underreporting, which is attributed to both denial and a fear of the consequences. Moreover, informal rules may be applied to medication administration, where actual practice differs from the organization's policies and errors are not reported because they comply with the standard practice (Smetzer, Cohen, and Milazzo 2000). As a result, the injuries actually reported are the "tip of the iceberg" rather than an accurate account of the errors actually occurring.

Factors that have been identified as contributing to this situation include concerns about confidentiality; the time taken to complete the report versus whether the information is perceived to be valued; the amount of information available on recognizing adverse events; and whether the reporter benefits or is punished for reporting (Kohn, Corrigan, and Donaldson 1999). Fear of the outcome also influences incident-reporting rates, including concerns of embarrassment by colleagues, patient reactions, and litigation (Leape 1994).

Human Factors and Cognitive Psychology

If the bedrock of adverse drug event reduction is a cultural shift, and if a thorough understanding of clinical and operational processes and hazard zones is critical to make change occur, the tools of the fields of human factors and cognitive psychology become indispensable in the design and implementation of systems to reduce the incidence of adverse drug events. Leape, of the Harvard School of Public Health, is a leading authority on the application of error theory to the field of medicine. His seminal work, *Error in Medicine* (1994), includes a concise and understandable summary of the implications of human factors and cognitive psychology in contributing to and reducing medical error. His article is as applicable today as when it was first published in 1994 and should be considered a "must-read" for clinicians and healthcare administrators alike. The main concepts from Leape's article are summarized below.

By directing the focus away from a blame approach to error prevention and toward a systems design approach, research into why human error occurs provides valuable insight for reducing adverse drug events. Human factors theory stems from the study of user–machine interfaces in technologically complex environments. Much of the work in this field has focused on the aviation and nuclear power industries. The field of cognitive psychology has yielded valuable models of human cognition that have been validated experimentally. Research from these two related disciplines has deepened our understanding of how people process information and make decisions (Johnson and Bootman 1995). Conclusions drawn from this research indicate that the causes of human errors are often beyond the control of the individuals involved (Leape 1994).

To illustrate the applicability of cognitive models in examining medical error, Leape presents a model of human thinking and performance originally developed by Rasmussen and Jensen (1974). The model describes three levels of mental functioning used to carry out everyday tasks:

1. *Skill based.* Both thought and action remain mainly unconscious. Functioning is regulated by stored patterns of preprogrammed instructions.
2. *Rule based.* Problem solving is governed by stored rules (i.e., "if X, then Y").
3. *Knowledge based.* This is the most strenuous level of functioning. Problem solving uses original thought that requires synthesis of both conscious analysis and stored knowledge.

Humans are generally predisposed to use the two less-strenuous levels of functioning that rely more on pattern recognition than on knowledge-based functioning, which relies on analysis and calculation (Leape 1994).

Specific types of errors are associated with each of the three levels of mental functioning (Reason 1992). An error of skill-based functioning is termed a *slip,* an unintended breakdown in automatic activity due to a diversion in attention. Factors that contribute to slips include fatigue, lack of sleep, emotional state, stress, and environmental factors (Leape 1994). An error in rule-based or knowledge-based functioning is termed a *mistake.* Rule-based errors occur when a rule is applied incorrectly to the situation at hand. Knowledge-based errors occur during new situations where the person exhibits a lack of knowledge or understanding of the problem. Many errors are not caused by human error but, rather, by complex interactions and deficiencies of the underlying system that are out of the control of the person directly involved. These errors are termed *latent errors,* or, alternatively, "accidents waiting to happen" (Reason 1992). Although, initially, it may appear that a person is to blame for an error, the actual underlying cause of the error is already present within the system. As such, the person is "set up" for failure by the system (Leape 1994).

"THE TALE OF TWO STORIES"

The National Patient Safety Foundation (NPSF), created by the American Medical Association (AMA), is a not-for-profit research and education organization dedicated to measurably improving patient safety in the delivery of healthcare. In December 1997, the NPSF (in conjunction with the U.S. Veterans Administration and the Agency for Health Care Policy and Research) sponsored a workshop on assembling the scientific basis for patient safety. The resulting report, "A Tale of Two Stories: Contrasting Views of Patient Safety," draws attention to the full story of the issue of patient safety (Cook, Woods, and Miller 1998).

The report underscores the importance of the second story that underlies each celebrated first story of medical error that is publicized in the popular media. The first story addresses blame and details regarding actions of the players involved in a specific incident. The more important story for the reduction of adverse drug events is the second one, which reveals the tight coupling of factors in complex systems that combine to produce systemic vulnerabilities to failure. It is this second story that points the way to effective learning and system improvement.

Critical to the way that the medical community, the media, and the public perceive stories of medical error is the concept of "hindsight bias," the tendency to analyze events from the perspective of their outcome. Hindsight bias often obscures postevent analysis of system performance. To truly make sense of these events and to develop ways to enhance safety, a more robust analysis of the contributing factors is needed than the methods currently offered by human performance research. Using human errors as the starting point, the "second story" concept reveals how multiple interacting factors in complex systems combine to produce systemic vulnerabilities to failure.

A discussion of second stories during the NPSF workshop resulted in the identification of common error patterns that could be incorporated into patient safety initiatives. Healthcare organizations can reduce the risk of adverse events by using available information about them to design or redesign their care and services so as to prevent the events from occurring in their own organization (JCAHO 2000). As a result of the workshop, the following conclusions were drawn from analysis of high-profile medical mishaps:

- Bad outcomes are the result of a set of factors rather than a single point failure.
- Enhancing safety begins with understanding the source of success as well as the source of failure.
- Research focuses the attention away from the people closest to the accident to an analysis of system failures.
- Research into safety helps to develop and disseminate safety research techniques that build our understanding of human performance and teamwork.

These cases help identify multiple areas for improvement that can be applied to other organizations (Cook, Woods, and Miller 1998).

Healthcare has much to learn from the aviation industry in terms of creating safer systems. Human factors safety studies began to focus on aviation safety during the 1950s when military aviation safety centers and the Flight Safety Foundation were formed. In the 1960s, the University of California developed safety management programs, and by the 1970s, safety management principles were incorporated in the aviation, railroad, and oil industries, as well as other disciplines.

These military-based programs were incorporated in civilian aviation practices, including the setting and enforcing of safety standards, accident investigations, incident reporting, and research on continuous improvement (Kohn, Corrigan, and Donaldson 1999). Additional programs were added such as Crew Resource Management (CRM), which focuses on training teams to cope effectively with non-routine situations.

Influenced by the work of James Reason, the aviation industry adopted the following precepts for error management (Classen et al. 1997):

- Human error is inevitable.
- There are limits on human performance.
- Humans make errors when performance limits are exceeded.
- Safety is a universal value.
- High-risk organizations have a responsibility to develop and maintain a safety culture.

The processes identified from the study of aviation errors observed that crew responses to errors included the following stages:

- *Error avoidance.* No errors occur because of active strategies and appropriate responses.
- *Error trapping.* An error was discovered and corrected before it became consequential.
- *Error mitigation.* Appropriate action was taken to lessen the severity of consequences after the error occurred.
- *Error exacerbation.* The crew's actions increased the gravity of the situation.

Through a process of research into the causes of accidents and an analysis of aggregate data to determine where improvements need to be made, the aviation industry has set a national standard for safety through the development of a knowledge base and the dissemination of safety information. The most important outcomes of this research include the development of a system analysis approach to error reduction and the identification of the need for cohesive, ongoing effort supported by substantial resources in order to maintain an effective safety program.

According to Gary Cohen, director of quality, safety, and reliability at the National Aeronautics and Space Administration (NASA), improvement in safety requires strong, clear, specific, and visible attention from the top of the organization. Attention from the top must focus on the following goals:

- Improved safety must be a specific, declared, and serious aim beginning at the top of the organization.
- Executives should make regular review of safety systems part of their work and schedule.
- A nonpunitive hazard and error system should be in place, with all personnel expected and encouraged to report errors and hazards, including near misses.
- Processes should be in place for the thorough investigation, review, and analysis of errors and near misses so as to identify patterns of hazard and vulnerable designs.
- Responsibility for oversight of hazardous systems as a whole should be clearly located in an individual with the time to discharge this duty.
- The organization should maintain an ongoing process for the discovery, clarification, and incorporation of basic principles and innovations for safe design, searching the healthcare industry and other industries and conducting research on human factors engineering, organizational and social psychology, and cognitive psychology for potentially fruitful concepts.
- Cultural supports for safety and its improvement should be reinforced continuously, such as thorough recognition systems for individuals and departments that contribute to safety improvement (Berwick 1998).

Research into human safety and the contributing factors developed in aviation have led to a cross-disciplinary approach to safety management that includes the concepts of human performance, cognitive psychology, and organizational behavior. This new approach allowed investigations of incidents to go beyond blaming individuals and, instead, to look at human error as the starting point for further research into system improvement.

CONCLUSION

As stated at the beginning of this chapter, the critical issues are awareness of the magnitude and cause of adverse drug events, a personal accountability to make patient safety a strategic imperative, and a commitment to move to action.

Patient safety has all the signs of an emerging technology: There are more questions than answers, there are no off-the-shelf process solutions or technologies that are "plug and play," and it will take old-fashioned leadership and hard work to get results.

Further, it will take successes at centers of evidence in the mainstream healthcare market with scalable solutions that are replicable. Such successful solutions are likely to be grounded in a cultural shift to prioritizing safety, to embody clinical and operational reengineering, and to apply the science of human factors and cognitive psychology. They will rely on products, services, and technologies to be "enablers," rather than relying on a quick fix.

It will not be easy to overcome many years of inertia and denial. However, it is absolutely critical that our administrative and medical leaders become champions for awareness of challenges, become personally accountable for making patient safety a strategic imperative at their institutions, and initiate the actions necessary to begin to have an effect.

Safety needs to become a core feature of our measures of outcomes, a factor into cost measures, and a key element to product selection and process improvement.

To those who are given much, much is expected. It is indeed an honor to be given the trust of our patients and their families. We have a terrific opportunity to take quality of care and safety to an entirely new level and, in so doing, to deserve that trust.

REFERENCES

American Hospital Association. 1999. *Hospital Statistics*. Chicago: American Hospital Association.

Bates, D.W., L.L. Leape, D.J. Cullen, N. Laird, L.A. Petersen, J.M. Teich, E. Burdick, M. Hickey, S. Kleefield, B. Shea, M. Vander Vliet, and D.L. Seger. 1998. "Effect of omputerized Physician Order Entry and a Team Intervention on Prevention of Serious Medication Errors." *Journal of the American Medical Association* 280: 1311–16.

Bates, D.W., N. Spell, D.J. Cullen, E. Burdick, N. Laird, L.A. Petersen, S.D. Small, B.J. Sweitzer, and L.L. Leape. 1997. "The Costs of Adverse Drug Events in Hospitalized Patients." *Journal of the American Medical Association* 277: 307–11.

Bates, D.W., D.L. Boyle, M.B. Vander Vliet, J. Schneider, and L. Leape. 1995. "Relationship between Medication Errors and Adverse Drug Events." *Journal of General Internal Medicine* 10: 199–205.

Berwick, D.M. 1998. "Taking Action to Improve Safety: How to Increase the Odds of Success." In *Enhancing Patient Safety and Reducing Errors in*

Health Care. Rancho Mirage, CA: Annenberg Center for Health Sciences at Eisenhower.

Bindler, B.R., and T. Bayne. 1991. "Medication Calculation Ability of Registered Nurses." *Image: Journal of Nursing Scholarship* 23(4): 221–24.

Bogner, M.S. (ed.). 1994. *Human Error in Medicine.* Hillsdale, NJ: Lawrence Erlbaum Associates.

Brennan, T.A., L.L. Leape, N.M. Laird, L. Hebert, A.R. Localio, A.G. Lawthers, J.P. Newhouse, P.C. Weiler, and H.H. Hiatt. 1991. "Incidence of Adverse Events and Negligence in Hospitalized Patients: Results of the Harvard Medical Practice Study I." *New England Journal of Medicine* 324: 370–76.

Centers for Disease Control and Prevention, National Center for Health Statistics. 1999. *Births and Deaths: Preliminary Data for 1998. National Vital Statistics Reports* 47(25): 6.

Classen, D.C. 1999. "Adverse Drug Events and Medication Errors: The Scientific Perspective." In *Enhancing Patient Safety and Reducing Errors in Healthcare,* edited by A.L. Scheffler and L Zipperer. Chicago: National Patient Safety Foundation at the AMA.

———. 1998. "Adverse Drug Events and Medication Errors: The Scientific Perspective" In *Enhancing Patient Safety and Reducing Errors in Health Care.* Rancho Mirage, CA: Annenberg Center for Health Sciences at Eisenhower.

Classen, D.C., S.L. Pestotnik, R.S. Evans, J.F. Lloyd, and J.P. Burke. 1997. "Adverse Drug Events in Hospitalized Patients. Excess Length of Stay, Extra Costs and Attributable Mortality." *Journal of the American Medical Association* 277: 301–6.

Clinical Initiatives Center. 1999. *Prescription for Change: Toward a Higher Standard in Medication Management.* Washington, D.C.: The Advisory Board Company.

Cohen, M. 1999a. "Causes of Medication Errors." In *Medication Errors,* edited by M. Cohen. Huntingdon Valley, PA: American Pharmaceutical Association.

———. 1999b. "Preventing Dispensing Errors." In *Medication Errors,* edited by M.R. Cohen. Huntingdon Valley, PA: American Pharmaceutical Association.

Cook, R.I., D.D. Woods, and C. Miller. 1998. "A Tale of Two Stories: Contrasting Views of Patient Safety." Report from a Workshop on Assembling the Scientific Basis for Progress on Patient Safety. Chicago: National Health Care Safety Council of the National Patient Safety Foundation at the American Medical Association.

Cousins, D.D. 1995. "Preventing Medication Errors." *U.S. Pharmacist* 20(8): 70–75.

Davis, N.M., and M.R. Cohen. 1994. "Ten Steps for Ensuring Dispensing Accuracy." *American Pharmacy* NS34 (7): 22–23.

Evans, R.S., S.L. Pestotnik, D.C. Classen, et al. 1998. "A Computer-assisted Management Program for Antibiotics and Other Antiinfective Agents." *New England Journal of Medicine* 338: 232–8.

Ferraco, K., and P.L. Spath. 1999. "Measuring Performance of High-Risk Processes." In *Error Reduction in Health Care, A Systems Approach to Improving Patient Safety,* edited by P.L. Spath. San Francisco: Jossey-Bass.

Flynn, E.A., and K.N. Barker. 2000. "Medication Error Research." In *Medication Errors,* edited by M. Cohen. Huntingdon Valley, PA: American Pharmaceutical Association.

Helmreich, R.L., and A.C. Merrit. 1998. *Culture at Work in Aviation and Medicine, National, Organization and Professional Influences.* Hants, England: Ashgate Publishing Ltd.

Institute for Safe Medication Practices. 1998. "Placing Limits on Drug Inventory Minimizes Errors with Automated Dispensing Equipment." *ISMP Medication Safety Alert!* Available online at URL: http://www.ismp.org /MSAarticles/Limits.html.

————. 1999. "Survey of Automated Dispensing Shows Need for Practice Improvements and Safer System Design." *ISMP Medication Safety Alert!* Available online: http://www.ismp.org/MSAarticles/Limits.html.

Institute of Medicine. 2001a. "Crossing the Quality Chasm: A New Health System for the 21st Century." National Academy Press. Washington, D.C.

————. 2001b. "Envisioning the National Health Care Quality Report." National Academy Press. Washington, D.C.

————. 1999. "To Err is Human: Building A Safer Health System." National Academy Press. Washington, D.C.

Johnson, J.A., and J.L. Bootman. 1995. "Drug-related Morbidity and Mortality: A Cost of Illness Model." *Archives of Internal Medicine* 155: 1949–56.

Joint Commission on Accreditation of Healthcare Organizations. 2000. *2000 Hospital Accreditation Standards.* Oakbrook, IL: Joint Commission on Accreditation of Healthcare Organizations.

Kohn, L.T., J.M. Corrigan, and M.S. Donaldson (eds.). 1999. *To Err is Human: Building a Safer Health System.* Washington, D.C.: National Academy Press.

Leape, L. 2000. "Can We Make Health Care Safe?" In *Reducing Medical Errors and Improving Patient Safety, Success Stories from the Front Lines of Medicine. Accelerating Change Today for America's Health.* Washington, D.C.: The National Coalition on Health Care and The Institute for Healthcare Improvement.

————. 1994. "Error in Medicine." *Journal of the American Medical Association* 272(23): 1851–52.

Leape, L., D.W. Bates, D.J. Cullen, J. Cooper, H.J. Demonaco, T. Gallivan, R. Hallisey, J. Ives, N. Laird, G. Laffel, R. Nemeskal, L.A. Petersen, K. Porter, D. Servi, B.F. Shea, S.D. Small, B.J. Sweitzer, T. Thompson, and M. Vander Vliet. 1995. "Systems Analysis of Adverse Drug Events." *Journal of the American Medical Association* 274(1): 35–43.

Leape, L., T.A. Brennan, N. Laird, A.G. Lawthers, A. R. Localio, B.A. Barnes, L. Hebert, J.P. Newhouse, P.C. Weiler, and H. Hiatt. 1991. "The Nature of Adverse

Events in Hospitalized Patients: Results of the Harvard Medical Practice Study II." *New England Journal of Medicine* 324(6): 377–84.

Lesar, T.S., L. Briceland., and D.S. Stein. 1997. "Factors Related to Errors in Medication Prescribing." *Journal of the American Medical Association* 277(4): 312–17.

McDonald, C.J., M. Weiner, and S.L. Hui. 2000. "Deaths Due to Medical Errors Are Exaggerated in the Institute of Medicine Report." *Journal of the American Medical Association* 284(1): 93–95.

Occupational Safety and Health Administration. 1998. *The New OSHA: Reinventing Worker Safety and Health.* Available online: http://www.osha.gov/oshinfo /reinvent.html.

Phillips, D.P., N. Christenfeld, and L.M. Glynn. 1998. "Increase in U.S. Medication Error Deaths between 1983 and 1993." *Lancet* 351: 643–44.

Physician Insurers Association of America, 1993. *Medication Error Study.* Rockville, MD: Physician Insurers Association of America.

Rasmussen, J., and A. Jensen. 1974. "Mental Procedures in Real-life Tasks: A Case Study of Electronic Trouble-shooting." *Ergonomics* 17(3): 293–307.

Reason, J. 1992. *Human Error.* Cambridge, MA: Cambridge University Press.

Rebillot, K. 2000. "Tackling Medication Errors Head on." In *Reducing Medical Errors and Improving Patient Safety, Success Stories from the Front Lines of Medicine. Accelerating Change Today for America's Health.* Washington, D.C.: The National Coalition on Health Care and The Institute for Healthcare Improvement.

Runciman, W.B., and J. Moller. Australian Patient Safety Foundation. 2000 (publication pending). *Iatrogenic Injury in Australia.* Adelaide, South Australia: Australian Patient Safety Foundation.

Smetzer, J.L., M.R. Cohen, and C.J. Milazzo. 2000. "The Role of Risk Management in Medication Error Prevention." In *Medication Errors,* edited by M.R. Cohen. Huntingdon Valley, PA: American Pharmaceutical Association.

Thomas, E.J., D.M. Studdert, J.P. Newhouse, B.I. Zbar, K.M. Howard, E.J. Williams, and T.A. Brennan. 1999. "Costs of Medical Injuries in Utah and Colorado." *Inquiry* 36: 355–364.

Wakefield, B., D.S. Wakefield, T. Uden-Holman, and M.A. Blegen. 1998. "Nurses' Perceptions of Why Medication Administration Errors Occur." *Medical-Surgical Nursing Journal* 7: 39–44.

CHAPTER THREE

Accelerators and Inhibitors

To improve is to change. To be perfect is to change often.

—Winston Churchill

T HIS CHAPTER EXPLORES the factors that accelerate the reduction of medication errors and adverse drug events and those that have a tendency to slow improvement work. A concluding section outlines discussion questions for two executive meetings.

FACTORS FOR SUCCESS

Most organizational changes fail to achieve their full potential, and many simply fail completely. The literature is pretty direct in this matter. When the Healthcare Advisory Board analyzed several organizations that deployed reengineering, it found that they did reduce costs significantly—in fact, by a respectable 8 percent over six months. However, the Healthcare Advisory Board also found that organizations consistently failed to hold their gains, averaging only 2 percent of the cost savings—not to mention the effect on quality, culture, and organizational stress—as costs climbed back to previous levels of unacceptable performance (Caldwell and Brexler 2000). Another study observed broad-based failures in most organizational interventions. In that study, over 50 percent of quality improvement (QI) programs failed, as did 30 percent of reengineering efforts. The study further observed that 29 percent of mergers failed and 20 percent of information technology (IT) solutions underperformed (Maurer 1997). In probing for experiences among healthcare executives, these findings are consistent with their personal experiences.

The critical point is this: For any effort of this magnitude to be successful, the organization's leaders—informal champions, medical staff, and managers—must be schooled in the nature of the causes of failures, both broadly and within their specific organizations, and must plan for success. Otherwise, experience shows that the most successful programs, the best ideas on reducing errors, the best technology money can buy, and all the human effort that can be amassed will result in a less-than-expected return or even outright failure. Understanding the nature of wasted effort results from a comprehensive assessment of past quality improvement, reengineering, and merger activity with an eye toward constantly improving the system of improvement. The QI methods, reengineering methods, clinical path creation approaches, and project execution processes, which cumulatively make up the organization's system of improvement, are not often considered candidates for improvement as are other processes, such as medication management, hip replacement, or patient transportation. Yet, the way organizations prioritize, identify, and implement new ideas is a system in itself and, hence, should be subjected to continuous improvement analysis just as the medication management system or the patient care system is.

The Institute for Healthcare Improvement (IHI) team, including Don Berwick, M.D., president of IHI, Tom Nolan, Ph.D., and Maureen Bisognano, after extensive research and a number of successful deployments, points to three factors of success (Nolan 2000a):

1. *Organizational will.* Top management and all formal and informal leaders must possess the will to improve. *Will* is a not passive term. It implies solving what "keeps you up at night." It implies the ability to set a clear vision, plot a course to realize the vision, and constantly replot to maintain a purposeful journey. It also implies not allowing distractions or too many priorities to inhibit accomplishment of goals.
2. *Ideas.* The organization must possess an inexhaustible database of ideas, even if it means "stealing shamelessly from others" as some have said. More than possessing just a library of great things accomplished by others however, this means having a thirst to identify process changes made by others.
3. *Execution.* The organization must be able to implement ideas flawlessly.

A fourth critical factor can be added based on experiences at leading healthcare organizations, the Juran Institute, and the Healthcare Advisory Board research:

4. *Hold the gain.* The organization must effectively deploy processes to retain the benefits of its will, ideas, and execution.

One way to illustrate leadership requirements for aggressive change is to compare the relationship between world-class athletic teams and medication error reduction teams. A perfect way to explore this metaphor is to consider what led the Chicago Bulls to unprecedented dominance in the NBA during the mid-1990s.

Throughout most of the 1990s, the Chicago Bulls not only were perennial NBA winners, but they also dominated the sport in almost all categories. Although the team's success is almost always initially attributed to Michael Jordan, as we shall see below, its dominance was the result of more than just the performance of a single star. In fact, the sport and that particular team provide vital lessons about winning, leadership, motivation, teamwork, planning, assessment, and measurement, and almost every other major facet of managing for aggressive change.

What were the factors that drove the Chicago Bulls to world dominance? The most consistent theories are:

- having a star performer (Michael Jordan);
- building passion around a common aim—winning;
- planning to win;
- organizing the game plan around team core competencies, not the other way around;
- playing as a team, not a collection of talented people;
- ensuring constancy of leadership and team membership;
- adopting a "We can do anything" mentality;
- ensuring that each member of the team—not just the coach—holds others accountable;
- letting only the best performers play, trading all others;
- not accepting mistakes and working toward flawless execution;
- following the rule of "practice, practice, practice";
- achieving superior performance through an attraction theory versus a punishment mind-set; and
- striving for constant improvement.

How does the way basketball is organized influence success?

- There is a way to keep score.
- The scoreboard offers constant and immediate feedback.
- Frequent time-outs and halftime allow the team to assess mistakes and correct them.

- The speed of decisions and actions is critical.
- You can do only one thing in a basketball arena—play basketball. There are no distractions.

ACCELERATORS

How might these lessons from basketball be applied to accelerate or achieve world-class performance in medication error reduction?

Engaging a Star Performer

Let's not downplay the critical factor of the star performer. You may not enjoy the luxury of a Michael Jordan of medication error reduction, but who does? However, the effort may depend more on grooming and supporting your Michael Jordan than you might think. Unfortunately, we often assign projects of this nature to any available staffperson or, more likely, to our only Michael Jordan, who is trying to juggle ten other critical projects simultaneously. Such a mind-set, though understandable, deserves considerable thought.

Every successful effort, whether in basketball or any other activity, seems to require the presence of a star performer—someone who, in addition to strong management and leadership skills, possesses a passion to excel. The aggressive reduction of adverse drug events and medication errors will rest on the shoulders of a dependable leader constantly faced with frontline issues. The successful champion must:

- have knowledge of the core process of medication management, including pharmacy operations, clinical pharmacology, quality management, some sense of the organization's IT infrastructure, and nursing care processes.
- have a history of getting things done. This is not a task for an unproven executive. If not someone on the executive team, this person needs to be someone with a track record of gaining consensus among department manager colleagues.
- exhibit persistence and patience. Some of the changes that are necessary will, in fact, require a change in the belief systems of physicians, pharmacists, and nurses about the best way to deliver care. Belief systems are difficult to evolve and may take years to change, just as they did in the automobile and other industries that achieved success in the quality arena.
- be a visionary and an entrepreneur—someone who thinks "big," believes "big," and can achieve "big." Some managers think big

thoughts, and some managers think of all the reasons why "big" cannot be achieved. The magnitude of this task requires a manager who sees every barrier as a fun challenge, a "what if we try this approach" solutions thinker. Never assign a manager who always says, "That will not work because...."

Building Passion Around a Common Aim

The notion of building passion around a common aim requires attention to several factors, each complex in its own way. The two most important factors are (1) the presence of a belief system or a culture with an intolerance for errors in the system of care; and (2) widespread adoption of a vision specific to patient safety and medication errors.

Presence of an Organizational Belief System

The presence of a belief system or culture that considers errors as intolerable events is essential. In the 1990s, the Chicago Bulls certainly possessed such a belief system—a set of cultural values, behaviors, and internal expectations of performance that required each player, each coach, and each support staff member to perform without deficiency and without error and to work as a team toward system perfection. Observers frequently laughed at Dennis Rodman's flamboyant behavior—coloring his hair, wearing wedding dresses in public, his crazy stunts. However, when Rodman hit the court, he was there for one purpose and one purpose only—to play his role flawlessly, with no mistakes, no errors, and no lack of focus. Despite his antics, the Bulls' belief system propelled him, night after night, play after play to excellence. Rodman's performance on other teams, although good, was never world-class.

As anyone who has ever visited a college football locker room can attest, the atmosphere is almost tangible. During its first national championship season in 1951, one strong image prevailed in the University of Tennessee's locker room. On the entrance wall, painted in large letters, was "The team that makes the fewest mistakes wins." Vince Lombardi, the legendary Green Bay Packers coach, inculcated his coaches and players with similar beliefs, such as "Mistakes decide ballgames" and "The only thing that can beat you is yourself." These expressions of beliefs, perhaps thought of as sophomoric by many, were intended to indoctrinate and standardize a culture around accomplishment of what they had set out to do: win.

In their landmark work *Built to Last*, Jim Collins and Jerry Porras (1994) listed what they termed *core values* as one of the most critical themes found in those companies that have survived decades of change while others disappeared. Core values are the composite set of corporately and individually internalized beliefs that sustain the organization through hard times and periods of chaotic growth and change. The authors observed five common factors worthy of note:

1. the presence of what they called "Big, Hairy, Audacious Goals," or BHAGS;
2. a cultlike culture;
3. evidence of trying multiple ideas and keeping the ones that work;
4. dependence on homegrown management; and
5. the belief that "Good enough never is."

The importance of the organization's belief system, as it relates to medication error reduction, was further supported in a recent meeting of colleagues at IHI, when belief systems emerged as one of four or five critical success factors to radically decrease adverse drug events. Jim Espinosa, an emergency department physician, would-be anthropologist, and leading thinker in the discipline of idealized design, characterized the organizational belief system as perhaps the greatest challenge of all. His thesis is that healthcare providers and leaders have come to accept errors as a necessary by-product of the very complex system of delivering care.

To transform a belief system, we must first deploy a framework under which we can understand our current belief system and our desired future state. That is, what is our current set of values regarding errors? Beliefs? How do our leaders and "heroes" behave when errors occur? According to Espinosa, in searching for an understanding of our current belief system and desired future belief system, we should probe for certain roles and frames of reference. Who are our heroes? What is our duty as it relates to errors? What level of error reduction do we believe is possible? Are errors part of everyday life or an "evil" to be conquered? Once we understand our current state, we can envision the way we think it should be. After we have identified the future state, we can embrace it and discuss complexities of transformation, priority areas, interventions that might move us in the right direction, and interventions to acknowledge and reward demonstration of the new behaviors. Figure 3.1 illustrates this construct.

Espinosa's discussion prompted some conclusions regarding the desired future belief system in which errors are miniscule:

- The heroes of the organization are safety innovators, formal and informal leaders who root out errors and anguish until the causes of errors are understood and resolved.

FIGURE 3.1. BELIEF SYSTEM TRANSFORMATION MODEL

Is Beliefs ➤ *"Future," Desired* ➤ *Interventions*

Beliefs

- It is a widespread belief, evidenced through behaviors of physicians, residents, nurses, and staff, that it is their duty and responsibility to report errors and energetically participate in efforts to reduce them. This idea that errors can and should be continuously reduced is further supported in research by Tom Nolan, in which he compared the factors of safe systems existing in other industries (Collins and Porras 1994).
- The organization must believe that "zero errors" are possible.

Sisters of the Sorrowful Mother (SSM) St. Mary's Medical Center, in Madison, Wisconsin, was another early adopter of strategic intensity in medication error reduction. As part of CEO Sister Mary Jean Ryan's quest for SSM to become the first U.S. health system to receive the prestigious Baldrige National Quality Award (which they were rewarded in 1999 as the first U.S. health system in history to receive a site visit by the examiner team), St. Mary's was encouraged to tackle this critical area of medication error reduction. Joining IHI's Breakthrough Series in 1998 to reduce adverse drug events, an initial aim was to improve the start times of first-dose antibiotics by 50 percent. Within five months, they had improved performance in this process by 67 percent and had instituted a process to replicate their interventions within 14 patient care areas (Anderson 2000). St. Mary's key stakeholders initially cringed at the aggressive goal of 50 percent improvement in such a short period of time. Yet, as has been found by those we interviewed, as well as in studies of other industries, the establishment of stretch goals is a factor present in most aggressive improvement initiatives.

As a first step, we would encourage all organizations to engage in an exercise to uncover their current and desired future states. Organizations should visibly post these states on flip charts at strategic planning meetings and take periodic internal polls regarding progress. In addition, they should plot their progress over time. This exercise can go a long way toward mobilizing the energy that will be required to innovate in the area of medication error reduction. Such an exercise would produce something like the following:

"Is" State	Desired State
1. Not that big a problem.	1. All leaders see safety as a critical feature of all system/process performance.
2. Not my problem.	2. Safety is our secret weapon. As an example, one of the best case studies we undertook in preparation of this book was of CareGroup in Boston. Jim Reinertsen, M.D., CEO, has declared that CareGroup will be the safest place in the world to receive medications.
3. Someone is to blame.	3. The patient is an important part of the care process and should be engaged in safety systems.
4. Errors are an unavoidable output of care processes.	4. To be error free is an achievable and desirable goal.
5. Admitting an error is shameful. Reporting an error by someone else is "ratting."	5. "Thank God, another error to fix." A culture of continuous improvement, supported by aggressive discovery processes.
6. Physicians are the center of the care system.	6. Error reporting and correction is honorable. (Ron Preiss, a consultant with Health Care Concepts in Austin and former Navy pilot, explained to us recently that the culture among pilots is that error reporting is considered a duty, honor, and obligation to the broader family of pilots.)
7. Fixing the problem will cost too much money.	7. Productivity improves as quality and error reduction goes down. This, of course, was a major tenet of the teachings of Deming and Juran.
8. Heroes are those who make the most noise.	8. Heroes are those physicians, nurses, executives, and staff who identify and fix errors.

Organization Vision Incorporates Patient Safety

The second factor in building passion around a common aim is to firmly nest patient safety in the organization's vision. Widespread adoption of a strong vision, or aim, specific to patient safety (reduction of medical errors, in general, and of adverse drug events and medication errors, in particular) ensures awareness among all major stakeholders—governing board, CEO, leaders, physicians, care providers, support staff, suppliers, and even the community at large. However, we observed it in only two organizations.

Although most organizations possess strong vision statements, few vision statements specifically include safety. In his breakthrough work on small-unit management, James Quinn (1992) articulated six differentiating factors, the first of which is to establish a clear, concise, sound vision. As revealed above, CareGroup CEO Jim Reinertsen rallied his organization around the vision that it will be the safest place in the world to receive medications. Another organization worth noting is Commonwealth Health System in Bowling Green, Kentucky. After the CEO and upper management attended a leadership session on quality, costs, and six sigma improvement methods, they set a vision to achieve six sigma quality by 2004 (Nolan and Haraden 2000). As part of that vision, the CEO declared safety as one of his personal priorities. A third case study, Heart and Health in St. Joseph, MO, driven by CEO Lowell Kruse's passion for excellence, transformed its vision to inlclude becoming the "best and safest."

Vision remained a consistent theme throughout our research into the accelerators necessary to drive for heroic levels of error reduction. Russell Ackoff's study, *Re-Creating the Corporation,* suggests that the entire success of designing ideal, or safe, systems starts with clearly articulating the desired aim or vision of the system being reinvented (1999). In other words, for the idealized design team to determine the properties necessary to achieve the aim, the aim must be specific with regard to error tolerances acceptable to management. How many systems and processes in healthcare were created or redesigned using a measurable expectation of the degree of error acceptable?

Planning to Win

The Chicago Bulls planned to win; they certainly did not plan to lose. In fact, all sports teams invest heavily in planning, with a strong emphasis on converting planning into execution. The importance of planning and its link to execution has been made by numerous researchers of successful companies, most notably, Nolan and Ackoff. Both refer to their planning models as idealized design models and both possess similar steps.

Ackoff (1999) lists five steps in his idealized design model:

1. Create a mission statement that clearly articulates the end state, and in the case of projects to optimize a care process performance such as the medication management system, include broad expectations for error tolerance, speed, and cost.
2. Define the properties of the system that must be present to achieve the idealized design, as expressed by the mission statement. Properties are defined as:
   - general (an adaptive, learning organization with a culture of continuous improvement);
   - organizational design (centralized, decentralized, hierarchical, matrix);
   - management style;
   - people properties;
   - product properties;
   - marketing;
   - facilities; and
   - environment.
3. Create an idealized design, or "conceptual model," as Nolan calls it.
4. Determine the closest approximation of the idealized design that is believed to be attainable.
5. Identify gaps between approximation and desired idealized design.

Organizing the Game Plan Around Team Core Competencies, Not the Other Way Around

This is certainly true in basketball. Although it is most obvious how teams organize offensive strategy around the star, more subtle is the comprehensive strategy that takes into account each player's core competencies, each player's stamina as the game wears on, and the talent on the bench. World-class performance can also be predicted in industry based on the organization's core competencies and their alignment with the organization's strategies.

Although James Quinn (1992) lists vision as the first factor of successful organizations in his research, as most research of this type reveals, one factor alone does not ensure success. The most interesting notion is that successful companies seem to organize themselves around their core competencies collectively or corporately, not individually. One of the early knowledge management thinkers, Quinn suggests that this mind-set in what he calls "intellectual capital" may be more important than hard assets. He even goes so far as to suggest ways of accounting for intellectual capital on the balance sheet. At this juncture, it is important to point out that the concept of intellectual capital management or core competency management does not simply mean people skills. Rather, as has been observed by Deming, Juran, Senge, and others, the entire system—its people, their skill sets, the way they work together, the organization's management style, the things the organization values, the surrounding technological techniques and methods it deploys, and belief systems—comprise "intellectual capital." As an example, 3M organizes by "technology platform," dividing its workforce into technology groups such as the one that has mastered the Post-It® note.

In studying 3M, Sony, Nike, Genentech, Apple, Polaroid, and others, Quinn noted that these organizations first focused on their core competencies, then on their markets and products, rather than the traditional view of market assessment first followed by strategy, tactics, and planning. Generally, the last property of the organization to be considered (if it is considered at all) is the collective core competency, or intellectual capital. It was further noted that many strategies in these companies do not aim to optimize economies of scale through market share growth nor do they view construction of vertically integrated structures, as is the case in healthcare today with our passion for mergers and acquisitions. Rather, they focus on building on the few core activities upon which they can exploit new markets and deploy new products. Stan Davis, another noted thinker on the new information age, also suggests that we focus on intellectual assets before all others (Davis and Meyer 1998).

Focusing on intellectual assets, therefore, would lead us to ask questions such as:

- What are we good at?
- How can we leverage these strengths into other processes, services, or even new markets?
- How can we leverage a relationship with another department, organization, or supplier to achieve some breakthrough?

To capitalize on this way of thinking, 3M sponsors inventors—7,100 employees with a $1 billion budget—who produce more than 600 patents per year (Gundling 2000). Most have no predetermined market or product application. After a budget for an idea is exhausted, management decides whether to continue or retire the research effort. Obviously, then, 3M capitalizes not only on its intellectual capital but also fosters an environment of great tension and pressure to advance breakthrough applications. However, mistakes are celebrated because so many, such as the famous Post-It® note, were blunders turned gold; 3M's library is full of such "mistakes." For example, one team intended to apply nonwoven technology into a bra cup, but the idea failed to materialize. Someone on the team suggested using the bra cup material in a surgeon's mask, then made of fiberglass extract. The concept became a huge success (Gundling 2000). This is a most compelling example of what is meant by intellectual capital. It is not just about people but, rather, the entire milieu surrounding a world-class team.

This forward-thinking approach is positioned against the traditional strategic planning model that leads to determining what market you wish to conquer or what goal you wish to achieve, and then to recruiting necessary core competencies to achieve them. Quinn does not go this far, but his observation that recruiting individuals with key core competencies into teams has not proven to be a successful approach to strategy achievement. Rather, team core competency is the more critical factor and an organization has a more difficult time achieving it through recruitment of individuals than by building services and markets around existing core competencies. This, of course, is not to suggest that individual and team skill sets should be thought of as static, but that the foundational core competencies are a strong predictor of success.

Although too new to research, this may be one factor leading the heroic success of Cisco, which surpassed GE as the most successful company in America, climbing from $1 billion in revenue to $11 billion between 1993 and 1999 (Garr 2000). Cisco's approach has been to determine what core competencies are required to achieve its vision, then to acquire entire teams and companies instead of recruiting a collection of individuals into a new team. Based on Quinn's small-unit management thinking, the following approach would accelerate an organization's path toward safe medication management system design (1992):

1. Establish a vision.
2. Charter a deployment oversight council.
3. Determine technical core competencies required to achieve the vision.
4. Deploy small units based on required core competencies.
5. Establish measures for tracking.
6. Agree on consequences for not hitting milestones.

How might we apply some of the notions advanced by Nolan, Quinn, and Ackoff to create a safe system for medication management? Perhaps by developing an aim or vision such as:

"To create a medication management system, from physician decision to order a medication to assurance that the patient has tolerated the medication as expected, that produces no greater than 0.01 percent adverse drug events per discharge, while converting 50 percent of error cost (cost and time saved in error detection, prevention, and recover) into cost improvements."

The following are our reasons for including so much information in this aim statement:

- The 0.01 percent goal is clearly a stretch goal, topping 3 sigma of 66,807 per million by 2 sigma levels. Depending on what source you draw on from the literature, the current level is somewhere between 0.2 and 2 percent. We have set a stretch goal that clearly will require "out-of-the-box" thinking.
- We expressed the goal in absolute terms rather than relative terms. That is, rather than "decrease adverse drug events by 50 percent," which is relative to current performance, we have chosen to express the aim of the redesign in absolute terms, based on the total number of discharges. Neither approach is wrong and both require the deployment of an effective detection system.
- We have bounded the process as broadly as possible to pick up all process errors and interrelationships from which adverse drug events originate.
- We have chosen adverse drug events in this example rather than the broadest set of errors or defects. Similar to the manufacturing industry's attack on worker safety, measured by "lost work days per 40-hour workweek," adverse drug events clearly are the most costly in terms of patient harm, detection, reporting, and recovery cost. Some might argue that the most effective and logical approach would be to consider all medication errors and near misses. This logic would not necessarily be in error but would lead to a broader set of issues.
- Finally, and critically important to the healthcare industry, we have set expectations for error cost recovery. The example aim statement suggests that 50 percent of error cost be converted into bottom-line savings (chapter 6 is devoted to this subject). Indeed, the issue of converting the cost of errors into bottom-line savings may be the only way to survive the massive cost pressures being placed on executives. The Balanced Budget Act, state Medicaid program cuts, and the failing managed care industry all are placing incredible pressure on the healthcare industry as a whole. These same pressures were applied by Japanese car manufacturers in the early 1980s when their quality and pricing forced the U.S. auto makers to completely alter their paradigms of quality and costs. As a result of that competition, today the American automobile is made with a hundredfold improvement

in quality and a tenfold improvement in productivity than it was 20 years ago (Womack, Jones, and Roos 1990).

It is beyond this example to delve deeper into the techniques of error cost recovery, except to plant the seed that establishing error cost recovery as an aim is important so that measurement, team membership, and creativity of design will be required to meet the aim.

Playing as a Team, Not a Collection of Talented People

The Chicago Bulls played as a team. Although Jordan clearly was the star and the "go-to" guy in almost every situation, those situations, especially sideline plays, involved critical actions by many members of the team to put him in the most advantageous position. Is healthcare so radically different in this accelerator?

During a discussion in a recent design team meeting, all agreed that, at the moment, most physicians believe that errors are someone else's problem and that nurses feel shame when errors occur because they have been indoctrinated to believe that all errors begin and end with nursing. It is part of our belief system and culture in healthcare that each caregiver operates almost independently and that "someone is to blame." Ackoff (1999) suggests a major idealized design consideration to regard people and subprocesses as part of a system. He states that parts of a system, as a collection of processes, subprocesses, activities, and tasks, cannot be operated on without loss of essential properties or functions of the system and that, when considered separately, system performance may, in fact, deteriorate. It is our tendency, in system improvement, process improvement, and comparative measurement, to "drill down" to find variation in subprocesses, but rarely, if ever, do comparative data consultants look to correlate changes in a subprocess with the performance of the system as a whole.

Ensuring Constancy of Leadership and Team Membership

The Chicago Bulls began to fall apart when Jordan took a sabbatical to play professional baseball. Many thought the downfall was 100 percent the result of his departure as opposed to a team dynamic, and perhaps they were right. However, what he took with him was not just exceptional talent, but also a part of the system of strategy deployment that left a bigger gap than just his individual efforts.

Many may remember Deming's Fourteen Points, popularized during healthcare's flirtation with quality and defect management in the early 1990s. The first point was, "Create constancy of purpose for improvement of product and service" (Walton 1990). Although this point addresses organizational aim, will, and focus, it also implies leadership constancy, perhaps in the same way that Quinn's concept of intellectual capital does. Many were not aware that Deming also constructed Seven Deadly Diseases. Two of the seven deadly diseases address the notion of team instability. "Lack of constancy of purpose" and "mobility of management" suggest that, in his learning, keeping a team together on a long-term basis is an important consideration (Walton 1990).

Adopting a "We Can Do Anything" Mentality

The Chicago Bulls could do anything, so mentality was not an issue. But what about those mere mortals desirous of a heroic improvement in adverse drug events and medication errors? At almost every course we teach on quality-based cost reduction, attendees make the following observations about the Chicago Bulls success run:

- Losing was never an option.
- The Bulls came to win, not to "not lose." Subtle difference, it seemed to us at first, but the more one ponders the notion of winning versus not losing, the more profound it becomes. In almost every sport, people can think of examples of teams that possessed a clear lead, only to blow it at the end. In many cases, such "come-from-behind" victories have less to do with the opponent waking up than they do with the secure team beginning to play not to lose instead of continuing to play to win.
- Status quo was failure. As Nolan (2000a) expresses it, "status quo is not an option" or in *Built To Last,* it is "Good enough never is" (Collins and Porras 1994).
- They set stretch goals. Jack Welch, CEO of GE, who popularized the notion of stretch goals and has been recognized by other Fortune 100 CEO colleagues for his strategy deployment prowess, credits the notion of stretch as one of five key tenets of GE's management style (*Forbes* 1997). So, too, does 3M, which expects at least 30 percent of annual sales to come from products introduced in the past four years and 10 percent from products introduced within the past year.

Ensuring That Each Member of the Team—Not Just the Coach—Holds Others Accountable

This was perhaps the most interesting of all Chicago Bulls accelerators, particularly when it came to Rodman. Here was someone who dyed his hair every week and even dressed in drag. Yet, on the court, he was a madman, 250 pounds of lane-hoarding aggressiveness who never let his team down. When he missed practice, it was not only management who jumped on his case, but his teammates. They depended on him, made sure he knew it, and made sure he knew when he let them down. That is the essence of "team."

Welch (1996) lists this as one of GE's five critical factors: "No one can be a bystander; get everyone in the game." Like GE, other companies have gone to great lengths to build "teamness," particularly within those indirect departments that do not directly serve customers. Some have even deployed service contracts in which service units actually contract selling arrangements with their internal customers (Quinn 1992).

In healthcare, we often act as though we are independent, detached parts, with little, if any, dependence on each other. But, of course, without recognition of interdependence, there can be no team and, hence, no team accountability.

Letting Only the Best Performers Play, Trading All Others

This is certainly a difficult one to process, but in basketball or any performance-driven sport, it is an expected and fundamental truth—players must demonstrate their excellence game after game, year after year. Moreover, players must demonstrate world-class performance before they are even chosen to be on the team, let alone play. Of all the accelerators that emerge during the quality-based cost course we conduct, this one creates the most animated discussion. We don't quite know what to do with it. In fact, the discussion generally concludes with the acknowledgment that in healthcare we not only have problems with concepts such as this, but we also have a difficult time with simpler notions of day-to-day, project-to-project accountability.

Not Accepting Mistakes and Working Toward Flawless Execution

To defeat errors and mistakes, it is first necessary to understand the nature of error. As discussed in detail in chapter 2, we know significantly more about the sources and underlying processes of medication errors than any other type of medical error. When considering only adverse drug events, an organization might experience only 0.2 percent of discharges from self-reporting systems, as reported by Leape, or the percentage might be as high as 21 percent if total medication errors are determined using multiple detection methods of self-reporting, computer monitoring, and chart review (Clinical Initiatives Center 1999; Moore 1998). Of course, in the medication error rate, encompassing near misses draws a much higher rate than the subset of adverse drug events. One study pegs adverse drug events at 1.8 percent of discharges (Clinical Initiatives Center 1999).

To determine the error rate for each dose requires making some assumptions that, because of the high degree of uncertainty involved, simply makes this an exercise for the sake of doing it. For each error per discharge, assume that only one error occurred in a subprocess (which, incidentally, is most likely a horribly low prediction). Therefore, in an organization with an average of 12 medications per patient per day and a five-day length of stay, the medication error rate per process step would range from 0.0033 percent (5.5 sigma) to 0.35 percent (1.8 sigma).

Taking the more realistic error rate reported by Jha (Clinical Initiatives Center 1999), the entire medication management system error rate is 210,000 per million, or slightly better than 2 sigma (308,537 errors per million), and approximates nothing close to 3 sigma (66,807 errors per million). As is discussed in significantly greater detail in chapter 6 on the relationship between organizational quality, error rates, and cost, most manufacturing companies would predict bankruptcy with an error rate close to 2 sigma. This is because the cost of quality (COQ)—inspection, rework, warranty costs, overhead to detect, analyze, and correct individual errors as they occur—would consume up to 40 percent of the company's operating budget (Harry and Schroeder 1999). In the manufacturing companies' estimation, the percentage of resources and staff performing indirect jobs, not direct production, would be so high as to make them uncompetitive (Womack, Jones, and Roos 1990).

As an interesting exercise, count the number of direct caregivers on a surgical unit and staff not providing direct care in a three-hour period. Add to that an estimate of the number of staff behind the scenes devoted to other non-direct-care activities such as inventorying, management, quality assurance, case management, supervision, and so on. Then, determine the ratio. What percent of staff is devoted to non-direct-care activities? If our error rate was driven so low that 50 percent of the inspections performed by case managers, risk managers, and other inspectors was no longer necessary, what would our non-direct-care full-time equivalent (FTE) ratio become?

Following the Rule of "Practice, Practice, Practice"

In basketball, in general, and for the Bulls, in particular, practice is the lifeblood of flawless execution. What is practice? It is repetition, repeating the same play under identical situations until all are exhausted and bored. Then, it is repetition of the same play under different circumstances until all are exhausted and bored. The importance of repetition is well documented in healthcare. Numerous studies by health planners support the notion that the number of CABG cases performed by the cardiac team is predictive of outcome. The Juran Institute conducted a study in the early 1990s that demonstrated for a national HMO that variation in outcomes in ophthalmologic care dramatically dropped after an ophthalmologist exceeded ten cases in a 12-month period (Caldwell 1998).

But how does a healthcare organization practice? In the automobile industry, significant resources are devoted to computer simulation of the effect of actual design changes on the production process. In aviation and space flight, it is the simulator. An emerging technology in healthcare is process flow simulation. Most common are emergency department, surgical services, and patient care processes, but little work has been demanded by medication management process owners.

Of course, in many ways, any Plan-Do-Study-Act (PDSA) quality improvement process serves this purpose, except that the tests are real, not simulated. The study step is intended to validate that the underlying assumptions made in the plan step are indeed accurate. Unfortunately, our observations are that most organizations do not maintain the same level of discipline as when they first initiated their quality programs. Many state that the PDSA cycle simply takes too long and prefer to skip that step in favor of implementing another change without the study step.

Achieving Superior Performance Through an Attraction Theory Versus a Punishment Mind-Set

Certainly, professional basketball players possess a call to greatness, and are appropriately motivated to exhibit that calling. To the person, they are not simply trying to maintain some minimum level of performance or recognition, or to retain the floor of compensation. They are always attempting to achieve greater heights of performance, and the entire system, including the recognition and compensation system, aligns to that mentality. Every one of them is an intense competitor. Dominant excellence oozes on the court. In part, this is true because of the culture of professional basketball. Much more powerful than the equally present pressure of failing is the recognition for world-class performance. And the excitement of the game simply magnifies it.

The very nature of the sport—from fans, coaches, media, and, ultimately, the players themselves—models an attraction theory of management. This is very different from healthcare in which most recognition and compensation systems are set up to reward "not failing."

What we are referring to here is a style of management, a new way of looking at how to drive superior performance as a result of management belief systems—management processes such as supervision and oversight, rewards and recognition, incentive systems, performance appraisal systems—all those processes that, in fact, make up the large system we call "management."

Recently, two esteemed U.S. senators and several policymakers hosted a small gathering of medication error reduction experts to discuss the best approach to improving medical errors nationally. Their first question drew an interesting response—silence. As potential approaches were discussed, they were asked to recall any successful government models, in any industry, in the past 50 years that had achieved the kinds of results they were seeking. Several minutes went by. All agreed that most of the examples were punitive systems that actually had produced less than optimal results and a significant waste of federal funds in staffing and bureaucracy. Moreover, these systems had consumed costs within the inspected company to prove that government inspectors were inaccurate. It was pointed out that among all potential improvement systems, attraction models seemed to have profound results, whereas punitive models seemed to waste everyone's time and money. In other words, stimulating improvement and establishing programs and policies that organizations and individuals wish to reach will achieve accelerated results.

In government lingo, this can be described as "supply-side" improvement. The Baldrige National Quality Award is one example. In the Baldrige process, organizations vie for recognition and distinction as a result of exceeding customer expectations for quality, safety, and cost. It is difficult work. Past winners, including Ritz Carlton, Ames Rubber, and IBM Rochester, have, each in its own market, excelled in all facets of quality, safety, and cost. Another example from the government is the U.S Agricultural Field Agent system, in which field agents are trained and then deployed to help farmers improve yields. They are seen as colleagues and educators, and are dedicated to the success of each individual farmer. How different from other government programs and quasi-government programs such as the Joint Commission on Accreditation of Healthcare Organizations (JCAHO), of which organizations are generally in fear. In general, nothing good can come from a government office visit. To its credit, the JCAHO attempted to create an attraction model with its "accreditation with commendation" approach. However, this program does not meet all the requirements of an attraction model.

Medical centers, IDNs, and independent entities can construct an attraction model, as well. What would be the result if the IDN Corporate Quality Office, with CEO interface, established a Quarterly Patient Safety Award? As long as the aim of the program, properly measured and following the other criteria discussed below, is met, individual departments and entire entities aggressively vying for recognition would, in fact, be on the road to world-class performance.

Successful attraction models:

- Make sure that the aim and measures will achieve the results you desire.
- Instill the mind-set that winning is the key. The program is set up so that everyone can and will win; the only variable is time. These are not one-time recognition events but, rather, long-term goals to be achieved by all. Some organizations will hit milestone performance targets this year; others may take longer. The Japanese Deming Prize is set up under this premise. Companies line up for years to be recognized.
- Establish several levels of achievement, something like Bronze, Gold, and Platinum. Set the bar so that 75 percent can win the lowest level of achievement and 10 percent the highest level.
- Focus the celebration on the winners, not the losers. You do not need to single out the losers (they will be in enough pain).

Performance appraisal concepts also play an important role and, unfortunately under present constructs, not a positive one. Peter Scholtes, a noted expert in the field of performance appraisal, makes the point that an examination of individual performance ratings in the average corporation reveals that a majority of employees are rated above average (1987). By definition, in a normally distributed population in which the median and mean are the same, average produces half above and half below. More important, Scholtes points to the glaring absence of devotion to the development sections of performance appraisals. The greatest emphasis is placed on the rating portion, which has the effect of fostering an environment of "not failing." He argues that to encourage an environment strongly driven to development and improvement, ratings should be heavily weighted to accomplishment of development activities outlined in the appraisal.

Striving for Constant Improvement

It is perhaps an unfortunate, but accurate, fact that most improvement efforts in healthcare have largely failed. Topping the list at 50 percent failure rate, substantiated by informal polls we have taken at many cost courses, is quality improvement (Maurer 1997). Following very closely are reengineering projects at 30 percent, mergers at 29 percent, and new software at 20 percent. If these figures are representative, the cost of quality, as discussed above, is unacceptably high. A presentation of these costs to management and the board, calculated as a simple accounting of all costs associated with full-time staff and team member staffing costs, consulting, training time, and cost, multiplied by 50 percent, would mobilize most to declare war on this form of waste.

Recognized for its innovations, 3M invests heavily in executive awareness, devotion of resources, and incentivization. In fact, one such management practice, the "15% Rule," allows staff to devote 15 percent of their time, at their discretion, to unassigned projects. To stimulate innovation, management follows what it calls the "Five Standard Wisdoms" (Gundling 2000):

1. Specific innovative practices can be imported into other environments.
2. Companies need to establish a "market-in " or "product-out" innovation strategy that fits the requirements of their market
3. The best way to foster innovation in a large, established organization is to create an internal "skunk works," an entrepreneurial unit insulated from the potentially stifling influence of regular operating procedures, systems, management personnel, and corporate culture.
4. Real innovation comes through a revolutionary breakthrough, or a paradigm shift.
5. Innovation is the product of strategic management actions.

Standard Wisdom 1 can apply to healthcare in that IDNs and medical centers might generate widespread acceleration of this concept by establishing recognition or even spot bonus consideration for those organizations, departments, teams, and individuals implementing ideas from other settings. Following Standard Wisdom 3, IDNs might announce the establishment of an elite testing unit and allow entities to vie for the opportunity to be recognized in this way.

Other industries generally follow the practice of separating design functions from production functions. SeaRay, for example, manufactures its yachts outside Knoxville, Tennessee, but designs them in Merritt Island, Florida. In fact, one of Ackoff's recommendations, in the deployment of idealized design programs, is to separate design from the production space (Ackoff 1999).

This concept, of course, is virtually impossible in healthcare, which is most likely the reason that product innovation has been delegated to device manufacturers. However, IDEO, a California product innovation firm, may have a testable solution. They recommend development of an innovative, creative, entrepreneurial "space" within organizations, where freedom to think outside the box is encouraged (Nolan and Haraden 2000).

Some healthcare organizations have established learning opportunities in which innovation is encouraged. Bon Secours Health System, an international IDN headquartered in Baltimore, hosts a monthly conference call of the pharmacists in its 25 facilities (Nolan and Haraden 2000).

Having a Way to Keep Score

In basketball, it is really pretty simple: The team that makes the most points within the defined time period wins. Period. In healthcare, it is not so simple. However, many believe that it will not always be this way. The Leap Frog Group, a collection of major manufacturing firms including GM and Ford, has declared that it will determine those providers with the lowest error rate and direct their employees to them. Until a universal measurement is in place, they intend to rely on process changes, such as the implementation of automated physician order-entry systems, to set contracting parameters (Conlon 2000).

In comparison, basketball coaching staffs also maintain a set of real-time predictors of success as the game presses onward. Measures such as "free-throw percentage," "minutes played per player," and "turnovers" are among them.

It is important to separate the importance of the detection systems and the improvement measurement systems. Detection systems are designed primarily to prevent an error from becoming an adverse event. However, an important exhaust of the detection system, when aggregated, is improvement information. Although additional data should supplement aggregated occurrences from the detection system to round out the error improvement data set, most organizations must devote significant effort to establish a detection system free of blame and fear, and that is easy enough to use so that error reporting occurs. Berwick (2000) encourages organizations to establish the following goals:

1. Prevent an error before it occurs.
2. Mitigate adverse consequences after an error occurs.
3. Improve systems to prevent future occurrences of system errors.

To pursue these goals, a viable detection system must be in place. Several detection system types exist, including those suggested by Cousins (1998):

- *Automated detection systems via an electronic medical record or bedside terminal.* The advantage is that no staff time is required to collect errors manually; the disadvantages are that the cost is high and integration challenges exist. Although expensive and complex to implement, industry quality improvement leader Intermountain Healthcare found that of all the methods it has deployed—early notification, drug allergy checking, drug interaction checking, standardized infusion, and automatic drug-dose physiologic adjustment—the comprehensive computerized system tops the list for greatest effect on error reduction (Classen 2000).

- *Voluntary reporting systems.* The disadvantage is that, of all the reporting systems, voluntary is the most variable and least effective. This conclusion has been shown by research conducted by the Advisory Board Company, Leape, Bates, and others. The advantage is that the cost is not prohibitive and best practices from other organizations can be incorporated into the existing voluntary reporting system immediately. According to Intermountain reports, voluntary reporting uncovers only 12 percent of errors (Classen 2000). As a side note, Intermountain also reported that available staff time—not fear—was the greatest barrier to reporting.
- *Audits.* Audits may be the most effective short-term solution. When combined with voluntary systems, audits have proven highly reliable and, when appropriate sampling theory is applied, not overly burdensome. Assuming a 95 percent confidence interval (only 5 percent probability that observed results do not reflect actual results), with a 2 percent precision, an organization with a 10 percent expected error rate requires a sample size of only 900. Intermountain demonstrated that small sample-size audits proved highly reliable and yielded error detection rates 61 percent more reliable than voluntary reporting methods (Classen 2000).

After the detection system has achieved a minimum reliability, whether automated, voluntary, audit, or combination, the aggregated information can be used to complete an error improvement information set. Frank Murphy, CEO of BayCare Health System headquartered in Clearwater, Florida, reviews the following data as part of his comprehensive quality measurement system (Murphy 2000):

- falls per 1,000 patient days;
- falls—significant occurrences;
- medication errors:
  -occurrences per 1,000 patient days;
  -mortalities; and
  -significant occurrences;

- pressure ulcer/decubitus ulcers per 1,000 patient days;
- ventilator-associated pneumonia infection rate per 1,000 patient days;
- bloodstream infections per 1,000 central line days; and
- CABG infections percent of total CABG cases.

John Berault, CEO, Medical Center of Louisiana in New Orleans (formerly University Hospital and Charity Hospital), has tracked selected quality indicators from all departments for several years, including preparation errors and dispensing errors. Preparation errors and dispensing errors as a percent of total drugs dispensed have virtually disappeared in the past two years, both dropping 97 percent from the high in FY1999 to early 2000 (Berault 2000). It was interesting to note from a review of the data, however, that the medical center experienced the same phenomenon that most organizations experience during the first few months of measurement: The error rate climbed significantly as detection processes were strengthened.

However, Berwick (1999) warns not to wait until the perfect solution is invented. Topping the list of "data detours" are waiting on the IT department; defining, redefining, and then re-redefining data needs; and measuring more than is needed to improve.

Having Constant and Immediate Feedback from the Scoreboard

In basketball, scoreboards are everywhere. They are in front of you, behind you, on both sides of you, with the biggest one over your head. They post the exact score, updated every time someone makes a point. They show the exact number of seconds left to play and post several key statistics in addition to the score. They have flashing lights and make noise. Even if you wanted to escape immediate feedback, you couldn't—especially the immediate feedback from the other players, shouted at the top of their lungs: "Pick behind!" or "Watch out for the $%#*@ on your left!"

"Okay," you say, "everyone knows that basketball contains a lot of feedback, but basketball is not management." What about aviation? Aviation processes combine a significant amount of feedback to ensure error-free travel. During takeoff, at navigation handoff points during flight, and during the landing sequence, controllers dictate a direction and altitude that pilots repeat back prior to execution. This feedback process assures that what the controller said is what he intended and that what the pilot heard is what was stated. Or what about manufacturing? Have you ever seen a sign in a plant posting the number of days since the last employee injury? Even the government reports the number of days since the last forest fire. So why is it that in healthcare we have not decided to post the number of minutes it takes to get a PRN pain medicine or the number of minutes to get a new IV?

Stan Davis, a leading strategy thinker for information age companies and author of *Blur,* suggests that successful management requires real-time measurement (Davis and Meyer 1998). Like a ticker tape stock report on the television screen, successful companies in the future will be able to pick off key indicators instantaneously. He asserts that it is no longer effective to manage any characteristic of the business—financial, customer feedback, safety, and business development—based on last month's data, provided halfway into the current month or last quarter's earnings reports. Rather, effective businesses must deploy sensors everywhere to gain immediate feedback regarding all facets of the business.

Visual controls, as our colleague Larry Abramson calls them, have proven effective in dramatically reducing errors in retail pharmacies. In a 1999 study of 24 retail pharmacies by the National Association of Chain Drug Stores (NACDS), a 68 percent reduction of high-incidence drug errors was achieved, in part as a result of the posting of visual measures and reminders about focus errors (Fleming 1999).

Frequent Time-Outs and Halftime to Assess Mistakes and Correct Them

Whoever heard of time-outs in healthcare? Why not? Jim Reinertsen, M.D., president and CEO of CareGroup in Boston, permits time at the monthly CEO meeting for attendees to share one story about a discovered error. One physician leader at Rochester General in New York hosts a meeting each Friday at which the team decides on one quality improvement that it can make before the following Friday's meeting and reports on the results of the improvement activity committed to on the previous Friday.

For several years, we have been advocating the deployment of a 100-Day Plan for tracking implementation results, as shown in Figure 3.2.

The 100-Day Plan is discussed in much greater detail in chapter 4, but its purpose here is to advocate some processes for early warning and correction.

Recognizing That Speed of Decisions and Actions Is Critical

Basketball—and, increasingly, healthcare—moves exceedingly fast, and evolving events are not surprising. However, when those events occur, decisions and actions must be made quickly or the game will be lost. Occasionally, events occur that are unpredicted and creative decisions must be made rapidly. What would happen in basketball if it took nine months for

FIGURE 3.2.   100-DAY PLAN MANAGEMENT METHOD

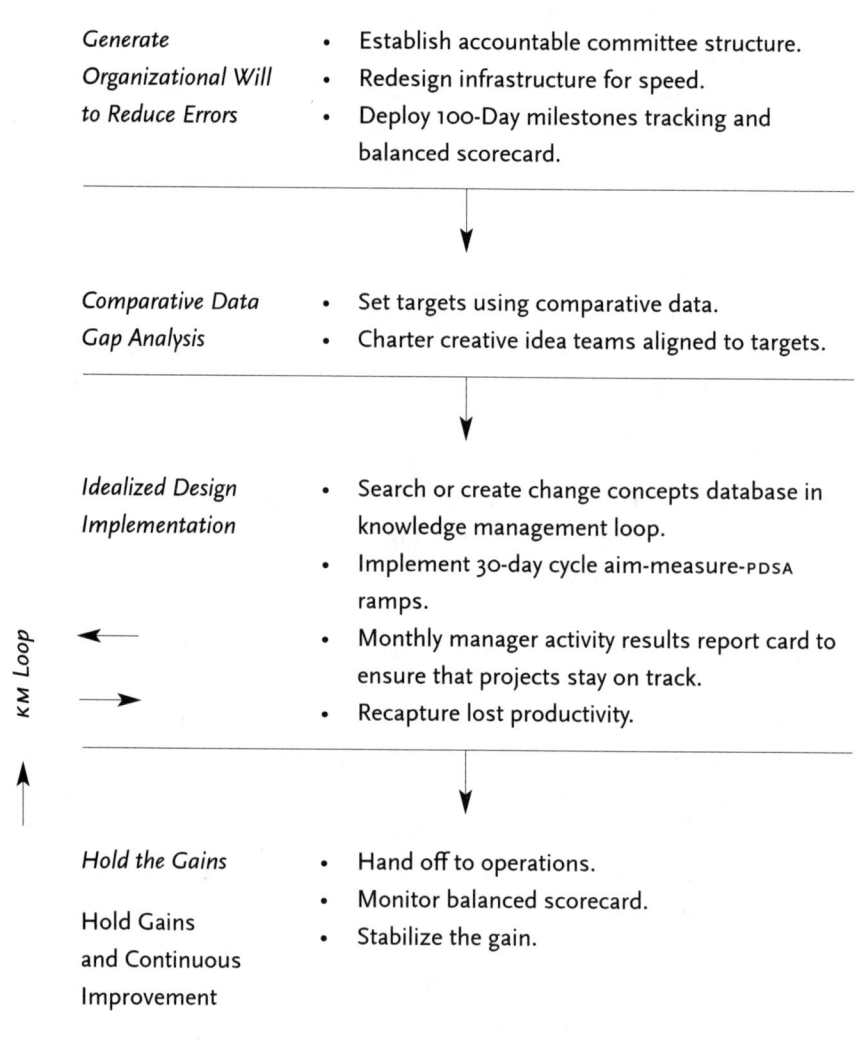

Generate	• Establish accountable committee structure.
Organizational Will	• Redesign infrastructure for speed.
to Reduce Errors	• Deploy 100-Day milestones tracking and balanced scorecard.

Comparative Data	• Set targets using comparative data.
Gap Analysis	• Charter creative idea teams aligned to targets.

Idealized Design	• Search or create change concepts database in knowledge management loop.
Implementation	• Implement 30-day cycle aim-measure-PDSA ramps.
	• Monthly manager activity results report card to ensure that projects stay on track.
	• Recapture lost productivity.

KM Loop

Hold the Gains	• Hand off to operations.
	• Monitor balanced scorecard.
Hold Gains	• Stabilize the gain.
and Continuous	
Improvement	

Reprinted with permission. Chip Caldwell & Associates, LLC.

a team decision to be made? Similarly, what would a healthcare organization be like that made critical decisions in two weeks?

Only Doing One Thing in a Basketball Arena: Playing Basketball

You can only play basketball in a basketball game. It's true—we have never seen anyone try to do anything else during a basketball game. In our work experience, we are often required to do so many things, often at the same time, that we are not at all sure exactly what we are supposed to be doing. One study (Fleming 1999) reports that pharmacists work under optimal conditions only 70 percent of the time.

LESSONS FROM SUCCESSFUL IMPROVEMENT MODELS

As a final note on the matter of accelerators, and as a check and balance of the basketball analogy, we analyzed those factors that seem to produce the best improvement results, most notably IHI's Breakthrough Series model. The following list emerged:

- quality as a business strategy organizationwide;
- aggressive, stretch goals;
- sense of urgency (The IHI mantra, "What can we do by next Tuesday?");
- management "firm intention";
- rewards, recognition, accountability, and consequences;
- disciplined methodology;
- measures of results linked to measurement of activity;
- idealized design change concepts, including the effective use of technology and standardization;
- use of subject matter experts to uncover evidenced-based change concepts and practices and drive credibility;
- enabling human resources policies (incentives, availability of information, focused training environment);
- entrepreneurial culture and belief system;
- comparative data for cost, quality, and safety; and
- holding the gains, or quality control, processes in place.

INHIBITORS

Those organizations that have made significant progress in the reduction of adverse drug events and medication errors are a distinct minority. Although we uncovered several organizations that are attacking medical errors, we found none that suggested they had attempted to convert the lost productivity resulting from errors into bottom-line savings. However, is healthcare that different from most other industries just starting on the quality and error reduction journey? Juran (1964) found that as far back as 1957, Peruvian farmers rejected proposals to double agricultural output because doing so would undermine the leadership structure in the village. Ten percent of the farmers elected to try the new method, which immediately more than doubled output, and within three years, increased to 75 percent. However, the remainder of the farmers still refused to embrace the new system of production.

Paul Batalden, M.D., one of the founders of the modern healthcare quality movement, observed early on that exerting organizational influence to change practices was futile in the absence of defined actions to prepare the organization to rise to a new level of performance. He termed this assessment *evidences of readiness* (Caldwell 1995). As observed by David Bodycombe, vice president of Premier's analytic functions, what we need may be an anthropologist, not more statisticians. Juran (1964) made the same observation. Culture, he asserted, is a "body of learned behavior, a collection of beliefs… shared by a group of people and successively learned by new members who enter the group." Therefore, behaviors, even disruptive behaviors, repeated often enough, tend to form the organization's belief system and require deployment of techniques beyond traditional improvement processes.

Barriers exist at all levels of the organization that distract our attention from this reshaping of the organization belief system. We recently assembled a focus group of four CEOS from among the largest U.S. health systems to discover barriers at the executive level; eleven emerged from the discussion:

1. information systems incapable of detecting and aggregating incidents;
2. lack of knowledge of how to convert error reduction into productivity gains;
3. insufficient capital for error detection and mitigation technology;
4. a "We're different" mentality at all levels;
5. individualist nature of medical practice;
6. fear and shame of reporting errors;
7. lack of effective feedback systems to detect, analyze, and redesign faulty processes and to hold the gains;
8. a belief that errors occur at "that other medical center";
9. comfort with the status quo;
10. the feeling that the magnitude of the task is too immense, causing immobilization, "analysis paralysis"; and
11. organizational disincentives. (An increase in one cost center to reduce errors in another cost center perplexes managers because they are measured and held accountable for their own cost centers.)

Further, Cabana (1999) sheds some light on our inability to effect process changes in his study of why clinical practice guidelines are not universally adopted, as illustrated in Figure 3.3.

FIGURE 3.3. FACTORS FOR BEST PRACTICE ADOPTION

Knowledge	→	Attitude	→	Behavior (N - 34)
Lack of Familiarity (N - 31)	Lack of Agreement with Specific Guideline (N - 33)	Disbelief of Expected Outcome (N - 8)		Patient Desires Nonguideline Course of Treatment
Lack of Awareness (N - 46)	Lack of Agreement with Guidelines in General ("Cookbook")	Lack of Motivation (Habit, Routine) (N - 14)		Conflicting Guidelines
		Lack of Self-confidence in Performance of Guideline (N - 19)		Environmental Factors —Lack of Time —Lack of Reimbursement —Worry about Malpractice

So what actions might derail an organization's efforts to consider medical error and adverse drug event reduction as a critical strategy?

1. The board, CEO, and leaders believe that patient safety and medication error reduction is really not their job but, rather, the domain of pharmacists and nurses. If they allow themselves to become distracted on this issue, grave strategic failures will occur because they are not focused on the really important issues—mergers and acquisitions.
2. Medical staff leaders believe that adverse drug events and medication errors:
   - are simply a by-product of care and should not be of concern;
   - happen across town, not here; and
   - should be blamed on nursing.
3. Pharmacists believe that adverse drug events and medication errors are their domain and they must protect it. Moreover, many believe that nursing and physician organizations want to wrest control away from them.

4. The organization believes that simply investing in new technology—a few handheld ordering devices, a couple of bedside terminals, and a pharmacy robot or two—will solve the problem.

5. Some believe that errors cannot be measured. There is too much fear, detection is messy work, and no one believes the numbers anyway.

SUMMARY

The introduction and continuous reinforcement of accelerators and the mitigation of inhibitors can have the most profound effect in the war on errors. Although additional solutions and solution sets will be created—some of them breakthrough—none of them will be optimized without careful attention to organizational issues important to any radical change. And make no mistake, many of the changes will seem radical.

REFERENCES

Ackoff, R. 1999. *Re-Creating the Coporation.* New York: Oxford Press.

Anderson, S. 2000. Interview with Chip Caldwell, March 13.

Berault, J. 2000. Interview with Chip Caldwell, June 23.

Berwick, D. 1999. "Lessons from the Institute for Healthcare Improvement Breakthrough Series." Paper presented at Premier Top Quartile Conference, Chicago, November 18.

————. 2000. "Reducing Medical Errors." Paper presented at Premier Governance Conference, Phoenix, AZ, January 12.

Cabana, M. 1999. "Why Don't Physician's Follow Clinical Practice Guidelines?" *Journal of the American Medical Association* 282(15): 1458–65.

Caldwell, C. (ed.). 1998. *The Handbook for Managing Change in Healthcare.* Milwaukee, WI: ASQ Quality Press.

————. 1995. *Mentoring Strategic Change in Healthcare.* Milwaukee, WI: ASQ Quality Press.

Caldwell, C., and J. Brexler. 2001. "Aggressively Reduce Costs While Improving Quality and Patient Safety." Presentation for American College of Healthcare Executives Continuing Education clusters.

Classen, D. 2000. "Detecting Adverse Events." Paper presented at Institute for Healthcare Improvement Medication Management Idealized Design Conference, Boston, April 27–28.

Clinical Initiatives Center. 1999. *Prescription for Change: Toward a Higher Standard in Medication Management.* Washington, D.C.: The Advisory Board Company.

Collins, J., and J. Porras. 1994. *Built to Last.* New York: Harper Business.

Conlon, P. 2000. "The Employer Response to the Medical Error Issue." Paper presented at Institute for Healthcare Improvement Medication Management Idealized Design Conference, Boston, April 27–28.

Cousins, D. (ed.). 1998. *Medication Use: A Systems Approach to Reducing Errors.* Chicago: Joint Commission on Accreditation of Healthcare Organizations.

Davis, S., and C. Meyer. 1998. *Blur.* Reading, MA: Addison-Wesley.

"Who Did the Best Job?" 1997. *Forbes* 159(1): 91, January 13.

Fleming, H. 1999. "The Human Side of Prescription Misfills Surfaces in New Study." *Drug Topics* 143(18): 16.

Garr, D. 2000. "Cisco Customer Satisfaction Systems." Paper presented at U.S. Quality Council Winter Meeting, Washington, D.C., March 15.

Gundling, E. 2000. *The 3M Way to Innovation: Balancing People and Profit.* New York: Kodansha America.

Juran, J.M. 1964. *Managerial Breakthroughs.* New York: McGraw-Hill.

Maurer, R. 1997. "Transforming Resistance." *HR Focus* 74(10): 9.

Harry, M., and R. Schroeder. 1999. Six Sigma, *The Breakthrough Management Strategy Revolutionizing the World's Top Corporations.* New York: Doubleday.

Moore, J.D. 1998. "Getting the Whole Story: The Way Medication Errors Are Reported Affects the Results." *Modern Healthcare* 18(51): 46.

Murphy, F. 2000. "BayCare's Quality System." Paper presented at Premier CEO Physician Leadership Forum, Tyson Corners, VA, April 18.

Nolan, T. 2000a. "Institute for Healthcare Improvement Breakthrough Series Results." Paper presented at Premier Rapid Response Forum, Charlotte, NC, February 17.

———. 2000b. "Widespread Rapid Improvement." Paper presented at U.S. Quality Council Winter Meeting, Washington, D.C., March 15.

Nolan, T., and C. Haraden. 2000. "Idealized Design of the Medication Management System." Paper presented at Premier–Institute for Healthcare Improvement Medication Management Idealized Design Conference, Boston, April 27–28.

Quinn, J. 1992. *Intelligent Enterprise.* New York: Free Press.

Scholtes, P. 1987. *An Elaboration on Deming's Teachings on Performance Appraisal.* Madison, WI: Jonier Associates.

Walton, M. 1990. *Deming Management at Work.* New York: Putnam Sons.

Welch, J. 1996. "Success at GE." Paper presented at Premier CEO Invitational Meeting, Aspen, CO, July 15.

Womack, J., D. Jones, and D. Roos. 1990. *The Machine That Changed the World.* New York: Harper Perennial.

QUESTIONS FOR A ONE-HOUR EXECUTIVE MEETING

Session 1:

Go to chapter 7, "Closing the Gaps" and select the exercise "Presence of Organizational Belief System" in section 1.

1. Conduct the assessment. Ideally, you will be able to interview each executive and compile his or her responses prior to the meeting. Study the results, looking specifically for areas of concurrence and areas of wide variation. Write these items on a flip chart prior to the meeting. If you are unable to conduct a premeeting assessment, you will be forced to break this exercise into two parts. The first meeting will be to conduct the assessment as a group exercise. Attempt to draw out in discussion areas where there is universal agreement and areas where there is doubt or variation in approach.
2. Discuss the desired state belief system. In a slide presentation or using a flip chart, present the results of the prework. Talk about those areas of universal agreement and those areas where doubt appears to be present and variation of approach exists. Record these on a flip chart.
3. After 50 minutes, summarize where you are and solicit "Next Steps." Request that a leader volunteer (perhaps you if you are on the management team), then chart some next steps to present back to the group within the next 30 days.

Session 2:

Again, go to chapter 7 and select the exercise in section 1 for evaluating the presence and absence of accelerators.

1. Have each member rate on a scale of 1 to 5 the effectiveness of each accelerator.
2. Ask for nominations of the ones with the highest scores, those that are working in your organization. Record these on a flip chart. Discuss how these accelerators became so effective.
3. Ask for nominations of the ones with the lowest scores, those that are not present in any significant way. Record these on a flip chart. If there are more than five, ask for a vote of the most important two by show of hands and prioritize the list.
4. Discuss potential next steps for the top five.

5. After 50 minutes, summarize where you are and review the "Next Steps" list. Have a leader volunteer to chart some next steps and present back to the group within the next few days.
6. Express the next steps as "aims" and deploy interventions. Chart the effectiveness of these interventions, over time, by repeating this exercise every six months and compare past, to present, to the future state. Celebrate gains, however small; create a sense of urgency to close the gap, however large.

CHAPTER FOUR

The 100-Day Plan

*So much of what we call management consists in making
it difficult for people to work.*

—Peter Drucker

THIS CHAPTER INTRODUCES a four-step process called the 100-Day
Plan that is designed to enable healthcare organizations to mobilize
for the discovery, reduction, and cost recovery associated with medication
errors and adverse drug events. As revealed in the previous chapter on accelerators, any effort of this magnitude requires a methodology that addresses several key features:

- Most important, quality as a business strategy must be the prevailing
  organizational mantra.
- The organization must recognize that patient safety is the ultimate
  tool to drive out non-value-added cost and to improve productivity.
  This has been the lesson from W. Edwards Deming, Joseph Juran, Bob
  Crosby, and others for decades, but healthcare has failed to appreciate
  that "as quality goes up, costs go down." Many healthcare leaders see
  error reduction as a necessary cost of doing business, not as the salva-
  tion of the industry, as did the automobile industry in the early 1980s
  (Womack, Jones, and Roos 1990). Whereas quality improvement and
  error reduction must be the driver, the exhaust is the combination of
  productivity improvement and cost reduction. The parallel effort is to
  recapture productivity lost because of time spent detecting and mitigating errors.
- The organization's effort should be clearly linked to its mission, vision,
  strategy, and governance and executive leadership priorities. The

organization and its leadership at all levels must be clear about the desired end results, or aims, of the initiative and must express them in written strategic documents. In deploying remedies suggested by Lucian Leape, the Institute for Safe Medication Practices (ISMP), the Institute for Healthcare Improvement (IHI), and others, the organization should work hard to ensure that these interventions are not seen as a project but, rather, as intermediate steps on the road to its vision. The organization's vision should be expressed in terms similar to those used by CareGroup in Boston. Jim Reinertsen, M.D., CEO, and his board declared that CareGroup would be the safest place in the world to receive medications. Lowell Kruse, CEO of Heartland Health in St. Joseph, Missouri, and his board have declared a vision to achieve six sigma quality. Envision the future state of six sigma quality and think backward from there. What would the environment be like if we achieved six sigma? How might we behave differently than we do now? What would the care environment look like? How would managers and management practices be different?

- Executive leadership consistently must communicate the desired outcomes of the organization's initiative; special agendas or disruptive biases are not present. If the stated aim is to "reduce medical errors by 50 percent and convert 50 percent of improvements into productivity gains in two years," executive leadership must be clear and consistent about the exact nature of their expectations, for example, of position control staffing changes or job mergers as a result of specific error reductions. The chief medical officer or chief patient care executive must not waver in his or her commitment to creatively adjust resource use, particularly staffing, as time is saved from error reduction.

- An appointed executive change agent should maintain accountability, responsibility, and empowerment to drive the organization's stated aims. Although most of the activity will be performed by key process owners such as the pharmacy director or nurse managers, to be successful the effort will require the leadership of someone in an executive position.

- Targets are stretch goals, resulting in the requirement that all process owners think out of the box to achieve the stated aim. It is evident to all that the status quo will not get them to the desired outcome. Creative tension must be present within the design teams.

- The change concepts database must be built on solid, evidence-based practices and championed by a recognized leader from either outside or inside the organization.

- The organization must execute a specific, focused effort to recapture lost productivity from error reduction. These savings will not materialize without deployment of match staffing to demand change concepts (as will be illustrated in chapter 6).
- Processes for holding the gains must be put in place for all significant process changes.

100-DAY PLAN MANAGEMENT METHOD

Over the years, we have piloted and tested several methods aimed at improving and accelerating results. A combination of those methods has been pulled together to form an approach we call the 100-Day Plan management method. This disciplined methodology has its origin in a strategy deployment process in which, rather than one-year plans, organizations break the tactical action planning process into three equal 100-day implementation periods, each followed by 21-day planning windows. The discipline is to implement only during the 100-day implementation periods and to plan only during the 21-day planning windows. In part, the 100-Day Plan method addresses one of management's Achilles' heels; that is, when problems arise, rather than redoubling efforts to implement, organizations have a tendency to halt implementation and to begin replanning, usually by adding more projects. This has the effect of postponing benefits from projects under way rather than the intended effect of increasing the return on effort.

In 1998, with the assistance of CSC Healthcare's Tom Enders, Tom Weigert, and Brenda Mounzer, Premier launched a new approach to process improvement. The method earned the label TopQuartile*plus* because Premier's foundation statement suggested that its major role was to provide its customers with enabling solutions to achieve top-quartile performance in quality, cost, and safety (Premier 1994). Tested in more than 150 engagements, the four-step model incorporated the success factors researched above and in the previous chapters. Finally, in late 1999, with the assistance of Don Berwick, M.D., Paul Batalden, M.D., Tom Nolan, Ph.D., Maureen Bisognano, and Carolyn Haraden, Ph.D., of IHI, the 100-Day Plan was strengthened by the addition of what we termed the *knowledge management loop*. The knowledge management loop causes the creation of a process-specific database of proven ideas, derived from subject matter experts (SMES). Adapted from IHI's successful Breakthrough Series model, the ideas within these process-specific databases turned into groupings of process design techniques that Nolan called *change concepts* (Langley et al. 1996). The importance of process-specific, evidence-based change concepts databases, supported by SMES, is covered extensively in this chapter. However, the importance of the knowledge management loop's inclusion in the 100-Day Plan (as will be discussed in detail in chapter 5) cannot be overemphasized.

The 100-Day Plan management method consists of four steps:

1. Generate organizational will to reduce errors.
2. Conduct a comparative data and gap analysis.
3. Implement idealized design change concepts and, if necessary, execute the knowledge management loop.
4. Hold the gains.

In step 3, the knowledge management loop is called to action in the absence of an idealized design change concepts database accepted by the creative idea team. The complete 100-Day Plan management method is depicted in Figure 4.1.

Before delving into the 100-Day Plan management method, an overview of its nature will help structure the process steps in the reader's mind. Its origin stems from observations by the Juran Institute that, when faced with inadequate results, upper management in all industries has a tendency to simply add more projects to its plate. Thus, management pulls valuable project implementation time to work on still more project planning, and the downward spiral begins. Often the effect is the suboptimization of all projects. This phenomenon is complicated by the fact that most organizations create annual strategic plan updates and deploy projects on an annual basis. In the current business environment, events are occurring too rapidly to rely on predicting 12 months in advance all that might happen. Therefore, the 100-Day Plan incorporates the following features:

1. Break the year into three equal implementation periods of 100 days each, called implementation cycles.
2. Nest 21-day planning cycles, called planning windows, between each 100-day implementation cycle. Using the basketball metaphor from chapter 3, the planning windows can be thought of as 20-second time-outs used to weigh the effect of implemented projects to date against the expectations at the beginning of the fiscal year.
3. Allow no planning during the implementation period, except for emergencies. As great project ideas are proposed during an implementation cycle, place them into a planning file for consideration during the next planning window.
4. Set monthly or biweekly milestones for each major project and assess whether each is on track, ahead, or behind. These milestones should be taken as an early warning system that projects are behind, placing your entire strategy at risk.

FIGURE 4.1. 100-DAY PLAN MANAGEMENT METHOD

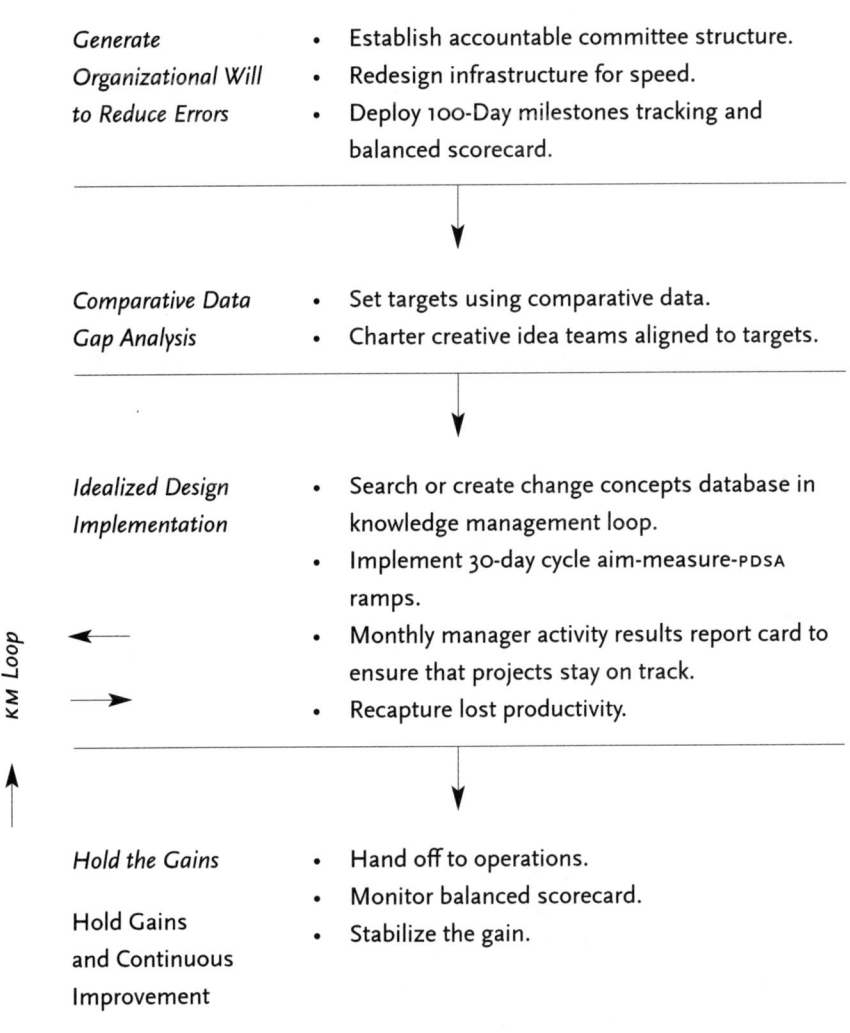

Generate   •   Establish accountable committee structure.
Organizational Will   •   Redesign infrastructure for speed.
to Reduce Errors   •   Deploy 100-Day milestones tracking and balanced scorecard.

Comparative Data   •   Set targets using comparative data.
Gap Analysis   •   Charter creative idea teams aligned to targets.

Idealized Design   •   Search or create change concepts database in knowledge management loop.
Implementation   •   Implement 30-day cycle aim-measure-PDSA ramps.
   •   Monthly manager activity results report card to ensure that projects stay on track.
   •   Recapture lost productivity.

KM Loop

Hold the Gains   •   Hand off to operations.
   •   Monitor balanced scorecard.
Hold Gains   •   Stabilize the gain.
and Continuous
Improvement

Reprinted with permission. Chip Caldwell & Associates, LLC.

Figure 4.2 illustrates how the 100-Day Plan process flows and where critical measurement processes (discussed later in this chapter) combine to form a comprehensive management system.

In explaining the 100-Day Plan management method over the years, the role of projects is sometimes confused. The 100-Day Plan is not a project but, rather, a comprehensive management system designed to establish the executive and manager infrastructure necessary to:

FIGURE 4.2.   100-DAY PLAN FLOWCHART

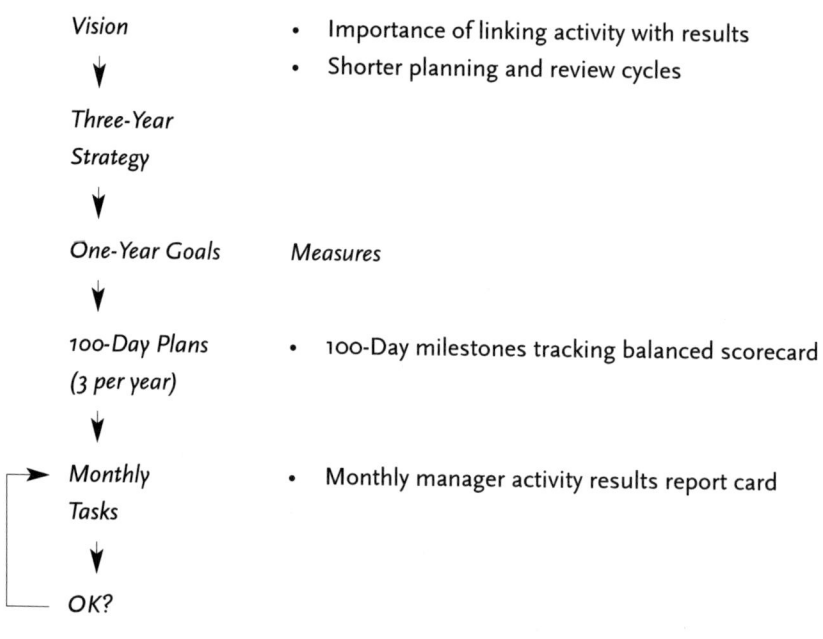

- achieve critical strategies;
- charter projects critical to success;
- measure results and activity along the way; and
- establish processes to ensure that gains are not lost after the strategic initiative has been completed.

Figure 4.3 shows the relationship between the 100-Day Plan and projects that might be deployed.

It is also worth noting that any successful improvement model is not sequential, although certainly some tasks must precede others. Instead, tasks should be parallel processed, wherever possible, to speed deployment to the desired end point. As the model progresses into several subloops, this observation becomes obvious in that, as one 30-day rapid improvement cycle nears completion, research for change concepts and appointment of the appropriate key process owners for the next 30-day rapid improvement cycle should be mobilized to avoid unnecessary downtime. Further, as several

FIGURE 4.3.   100-DAY PLAN AND PROJECT DEPLOYMENT

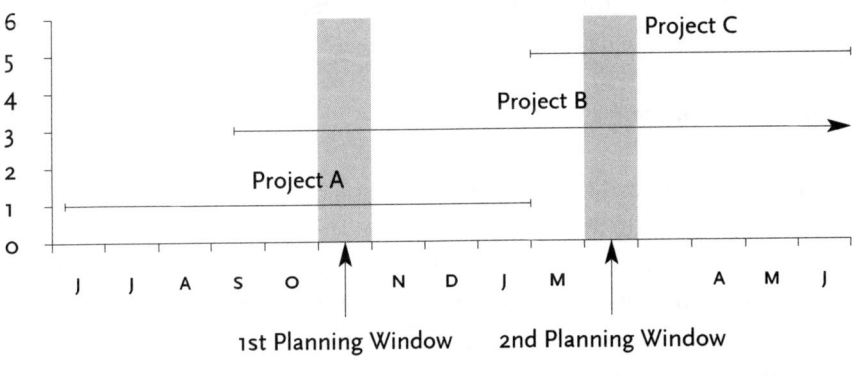

30-day rapid improvement cycles pass, "hold-the-gains" measurement creates another subset of parallel tasks. In fact, the "hold-the-gains" process evolves into the organization's quality control program managed as a part of everyday practice by the organization's middle management team.

STEP 1. GENERATE ORGANIZATIONAL WILL TO REDUCE ERRORS

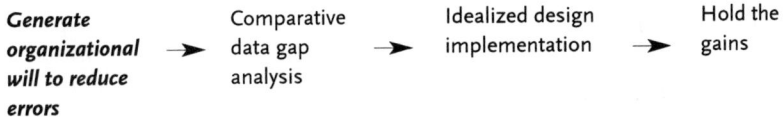

The first step in the 100-Day Plan management method is to generate the organizational will to aggressively reduce medical errors. As discussed numerous times, any successful initiative requires planning, preparation, publication of a precise aim, establishment of measures, and assignment of accountable executives, process owners and analysts, and resources. Three tasks drive the completion of this step. The organization must:

1. establish an accountable executive and committee structure;
2. redesign the infrastructure for speed; and
3. deploy a balanced scorecard and 100-day milestones tracking.

Establish an Accountable Executive and Committee Structure

The critical first task in generating organizational will is to set up an effective structure to drive the 100-Day Plan's four-step process. Several tasks are included in this activity.

Commit to the Initiative

The beginning is really the operationalization of the critical success factor that Berwick refers to as organizational will. It is not just individual will or the will of a handful of executives and middle managers but, rather, the collective will of the entire organization. Some refer to this as organizational culture; others, like us, refer to it as the organization's belief system.

Many of the organizations we interviewed, studied in the literature, or ran across in preparation for this book had little appreciation for the importance of the intense involvement of senior leadership. Outside healthcare, this is not the case. Consider, for example, Toyota. It is Toyota's belief that it is not only the job of senior management to lay out the organization's plans and strategies, but also to coach in the new methods of work. So strong is Toyota's belief in the central role of senior management that senior managers do not answer inquiries from middle managers regarding even simple aspects of their improvement approach. A quote from the senior leader of Toyota's Creative Idea Committee illustrates: "Every year we get requests for detailed information about our company's suggestion system. But when the request is made by phone and the other party's position is only a middle manager or a lower-level executive, we can only apologize for giving a mere outline of basic facts, and for declining to give any information beyond that" (Yasuda 1991).

Give the Initiative a Name

Every critical program must be given a "name" so that all key stakeholders can relate to the objectives consistently. Therefore, the first step is to name the initiative and articulate the scope and boundaries. Many successful organizations invest a lot of time coming up with cute names or acronyms; others declare that such conventions devalue the critical strategic nature of the initiative. It has been our experience that both are right. If your past successful efforts and current culture value such naming conventions, capitalize on it. On the other hand, as you reflect on past successes and false starts and determine that such conventions are present in those initiatives producing less-than-desired results, avoid flashy names. Regardless, the main point is to call the initiative something and to rely on that name to carry you through the first two to three years.

Give the Initiative Sizzle

It also has been our experience that every major initiative requires a little sizzle every two to three years. Thus, if you have had an initiative to reduce medical errors for some time, but it has become less glamorous, relaunch it or provide a little extra sizzle. Some may feel that such tactics trivialize the effort, but this caution does not bear up to our observations.

A story related in *Mentoring Strategic Change in Healthcare* (Caldwell 1995) illustrates the importance of sizzle. After only a few months into West Paces Medical Center's quality journey, the facility began receiving requests for site visits. Most visitors were healthcare executives interested in learning new techniques to deploy within their own organizations, but, occasionally, a non-healthcare executive would show up. That was the case when the CEO of a rubber hose supplier to the automobile industry visited. The company managed by this CEO had received numerous quality awards for its efforts, and the executives at West Paces recalled being very intimidated and a bit embarrassed that this experienced CEO had visited them at such an early and immature stage of their quality system deployment. At the conclusion of the session, the executives confessed their embarrassment, after which the visiting CEO conveyed a critical lesson. He advised them that every successful multiyear strategy requires frequent reenergizing to maintain momentum. As CEO, and hence senior quality officer, he was sensing a disturbing loss of enthusiasm in his own company and was considering instituting a storyboard process to reactivate his rate of improvement. The CEO conducted quality rounds, and staff were videotaped telling their quality stories, capitalizing on the "sizzle" to keep it interesting.

The lesson is this: Regardless of past successes or failures, the excitement will inevitably wear off. It remains the role of senior leadership to constantly be on guard for complacency and loss of momentum and, once discovered, to quickly institute a new "bell or whistle," regardless of how silly it may appear, to maintain momentum. West Paces was constantly on the lookout for new ways to highlight its successes.

Appoint an Executive Change Agent

Any effort of this magnitude will require significant commitment from a persuasive, accountable executive in the role of change agent. Although all the steps in the process are critical, the appointment of a change agent is among the most important. Generally, a manager at the level of executive vice president should be appointed unless medical error reduction is not a strategic priority. The executive change agent is supported by individuals within the organization who are knowledgeable about underlying core processes, such as the pharmacy director, clinical chiefs, medical directors, nursing executives, laboratory managers, risk managers, and quality professionals. In chapter 7 "Closing the Gaps" use the exercise in section II, step I to determine the characteristics of a successful executive change agent in your specific organization.

Conduct an Evidence of Readiness Assessment

To assess organizational will, it will be necessary to conduct an assessment of the current and desired future states. The notion of assessing readiness prior to the initiation of a major new strategy was highlighted at West Paces Medical Center by our mentor, Paul Batalden, now at Dartmouth's Center for Change Leadership. After observing a few failed attempts to advance our quality program to a new level of performance, Batalden asked us to seek evidences of readiness. This became important when we began to engage clinical practice changes and required physician collaboration, or when we sought to measure variation in critical processes and required statistical process control (SPC) knowledge at the middle-manager level.

A first task for the executive change agent is to understand the organization's readiness to aggressively attack the medical errors priority and to identify pockets of support and resistance. Chip Caldwell & Associates, LLC, has constructed a tool called the Evidence of Readiness Index (available at www.chipcaldwellassoc.com/resources) to provide this awareness. Organizations can develop their own tool or acquire an existing one. It is often advantageous to bring in an outside surveyor to interview key staff to avoid bias and encourage straightforward answers. For those in multi-institutional systems, bringing in an executive from a sister organization to interview your key staff and surveying theirs will serve this purpose, or engaging outside experts or consulting firms familiar with assessment of belief systems can accomplish the task.

Organizations desiring to build their own assessment tools might want to use the belief system exercise in section I of chapter 7. In addition to the assessment, the executive change agent, along with a team of trusted colleagues, should conduct high-level research into the nature and extent of the medical errors issue within the organization and within the industry.

Much has already been written about the problem, and asking leaders to react to some of these published articles will shed valuable light on their personal resolve and passion to join or lead the effort within their own spheres of influence. The scoping may come from an analysis of quality variance, compatibility and/or conflict with existing strategic priorities, presence of logical executive champions, or scarcity of resources, including lack of management resolve. It is important to understand and name these accelerators and inhibitors to fully attack the issue of medical errors. Poll executive, medical, and management leadership to gain a full appreciation of their knowledge of the seriousness of the issue within your organization and, more broadly, within the industry. Probe for their feelings about the priority of tackling the issue at this time, barriers to error reduction, and their own knowledge base of how to go about aggressive error reduction and what has worked at other organizations.

Having completed this, the executive change agent and other leaders will have some sense of areas to be addressed, champions from both the formal and informal leadership, potential detractors and their reasons, resources required, and so on. This knowledge is the basis for the next steps.

Build a Critical Mass of Champions

As a result of interviews and the Evidence of Readiness Index, you will have some sense of whom to recruit for the effort. Most often, the temptation, or even management logic, is to focus on the detractors in order to achieve momentum. For example, Batalden provided a critical insight several years ago when West Paces Medical Center was faced with a disturbing lack of support from its diabetologists. The senior management team anguished over its inability to recognize the strategic value of the quality initiative. We invested significant time and energy to "convert" the physicians, until Batalden suggested we refocus our time, energy, and resources on those physicians who supported our vision (Caldwell 1995). This simple redirection not only accelerated our results, but it also made our work significantly more enjoyable. We began working with physicians who shared our vision of quality, who supported us in our failures and cheered our successes, and who came in early and went home late.

Any effort of this magnitude requires a critical mass of champions from all constituencies, who must be kept in constant communication and constantly quizzed regarding areas that require additional support, bolstering, or acknowledgment. At this juncture, it also is important to identify any leaders likely to oppose your vision. Do not invest significant time selling them on activities but, rather, be aware of their potentially harmful presence during critical times and deploy countermeasures to mitigate the potentially negative effect they may have.

Another key step in generating organizational will is to mitigate as many impediments to progress as possible, ensuring accountability as well as effective rewards and recognition.

The more difficult of the two is accountability. It has been our experience that because of our desire to be forgiving, we overlook those who consistently fail to achieve objectives, and follow a "three strikes and you're out" mantra, which very often becomes a .100 batting average. Coaching managers through their successes and failures is an important skill of all successful executives, and no one would advocate an overzealous or harsh management style when it comes to ensuring performance. But an overly forgiving nature is a double-edged sword. While imparting forgiveness, a lack of insistence on world-class performance will ultimately lead to an organizational belief system that mediocre performance is acceptable, that failure without improvement is an option. There are several coaching approaches for performance that is consistently under par. The effective executive will:

1. Be clear about performance expectations and spell out precisely what this means in measurable terms. For example, "Our aim is to reduce adverse drug events and medication errors by 25 percent in 12 months while capitalizing on productivity gains from error reduction." Further, "Status quo is not an option, and a sense of urgency as manifested through each manager's implementation of one change per month is critical to our success."

2. Establish an effective oversight and review system that frequently records accomplishments of managers, both those who exceed expectations and those who are behind. The 100-Day Plan management method was created with this purpose in mind.

3. Be quick to applaud those who exceed expectations, but be equally quick to explore the reasons for subpar performance with those who fall short. Once symptoms are diagnosed, an effective manager will provide adequate resources and time to correct the current underperformance trend and will follow the corrective plan carefully by shortening the time for milestone monitoring. Further, he or she will rechart the course as often as seems appropriate and devote additional resources, education, benchmarking assistance, and other support, as necessary.

4. When it becomes apparent that the manager will not succeed, act quickly to assign his or her management responsibilities to another manager. Recently, Jack Welch, CEO of GE and acknowledged world-class management practitioner, advised a group of health system CEOS

on this subject (Welch 1996). It was his observation that management consistently acts too slow—in strategic realignment; in abandoning underperforming assets and programs, unsuccessful projects, strategies, and tactics; and, particularly, in making personnel moves. He observed: "Give Harry another chance. Six months isn't going to change Harry. Harry has been here thirty years, doing the same things. Six more months isn't going to change Harry. Get Harry out of the way." As harsh as this judgment may seem, a demand for high performance is a characteristic of most successful organizations.

As long as a process similar to the one proposed here is followed, with effective measurement and coaching, the effect of rapid decision making regarding underperformers helps to support a belief system that status quo is not an option and a sense of urgency is expected of all managers. An underperforming, overmatched manager is recognized for such by his or her peers long before executive management observes it. This is often a very difficult situation for all managers because of the discomfort caused by consistent acceptance of underperformance.

The same is true for the importance of rewards and recognition. Organizations have a tendency to socialize their champions—those who are recognized as heroes are often managers who communicate easily, tell their stories effectively, happen to be at the right places at the right times, and generally find it easy to relate to executive management, physicians, and colleagues. The heroes are not necessarily those who exceed performance expectations, time and time again, project after project, budget cycle after budget cycle. Often these individuals are less glamorous, do not seek public recognition, and may not be as outgoing in nature but, instead, prefer to let others dominate management meeting discussions. They simply get the job done.

It is important to design reward and recognition structures so that the real heroes stand out. Following are some of the more effective means of recognition we have seen (Caldwell 1995).

Storyboards

A technique proven effective in the mid-1980s by Florida Power and Light (and since popularized by leading healthcare quality leaders) is the visible placement of storyboards. A storyboard is a poster containing quality improvement project goals, data, conclusions, interventions, and results. (For more information on the construction and success factors of storyboards, see *Mentoring Strategic Change in Healthcare* [Caldwell 1995].) In the past some organizations made storyboard creation and maintenance a burdensome chore for the manager. Simplicity appears to be the best approach. Laying out the documents normally expected of a project leader—aim statement, trend graphs, flowcharts, next steps—in storyboard format versus a notebook that is rarely, if ever, reviewed by others should serve the purpose. Some might feel that "We've been there, done that," but dusting off the storyboards to illustrate progress, particularly if measurements are visibly present, can only accelerate implementation, learning, and recognition. Generally, when confronted by skeptics, our usual response is to elicit all the reasons why storyboards should not be used and all the reasons they should. The most frequent conclusion is that an organization has a lot to gain from storyboard use and very little, if anything, to lose. And as legitimate barriers surface, creative quality professionals and managers can quickly resolve them while protecting the positive features.

Creative Idea Committee Reviews

This once-popular technique deserves resurrection. Progress review sessions are commissioned monthly by the patient safety creative idea committee, as discussed below, or by an existing executive management committee. Strategic performance review, in general, and medication error reduction, in particular, should not be relegated to a department or subcommittee but, instead, should be visible to executive management. A typical review session lasts about two hours and contains presentations by four to eight managers. At the beginning of the session, the executive change agent presents the run chart or trend graph showing both error reduction to date and the cumulative number of monthly implementations executed by participating managers. Following this overview, each manager should be given no more than 15 minutes to present the results of the implementations since the last presentation and the cumulative trend line of error reduction for the particular function. It is not usually effective to bring in the entire team and show detailed flowcharts and specifics of the team's work. Instead, focus only on two factors—what process changes have been implemented since this manager's last review, and what the trend line graph shows in terms of results in decreased errors.

Storyboard Reviews

Another form of recognition features a quarterly storyboard review session, voluntarily attended by the entire organization, at which participating managers place their storyboards around an auditorium, cafeteria, or other room suitable for this purpose. The session generally lasts two hours, and light refreshments might be served. Hosting a session just prior to a quarterly medical staff meeting might draw attention and recognition from medical staff leaders.

CEO Rounds

A technique that ensures the appropriate level of CEO awareness is a quarterly tour of storyboards. Informality is generally the best approach, and some CEOS make notes and comments to the manager and/or team. Sister Mary Jean Ryan, CEO of the SSM Health System headquartered in St. Louis (and the first health system to be distinguished by the Baldrige National Quality Award Committee with a site visit in 1999) hosts a Gratitude Tour, in which she tours each facility to acknowledge the facility's efforts in error reduction and quality improvement (Ryan 2000).

The Good Idea Club

Taken from the Toyota Suggestion System, the Good Idea Club is an acknowledgment award granted to teams and individuals for implemented innovations (Yasuda 1991). The ideas need not be glamorous or magnificent but, rather, of substantial benefit or frequency. A central feature of the Good Idea Club is that creative idea teams review each implemented idea and award various recognitions depending on the category. Although we would not advocate individual awards, which have a tendency to stimulate individual competition and thwart teamwork, we strongly support recognition efforts such as the Good Idea Club. Adapted for medication error initiatives, possible categories for team awards might include "most effect on medication error reduction" or "most implemented ideas."

Staff Newsletters and News Releases

Recognizing accomplishments, organizationwide and by specific managers and teams—in employee newsletters, Intranet sites, community news releases, and other forms of public recognition—goes a long way toward keeping the initiative in front of key constituency groups and acknowledging the work to date.

Merit Reviews

Error reduction and implementation of monthly process changes should become components of every manager's performance review. If bonuses are in place, a high percentage should be allocated to error reduction and monthly activity.

Awards Programs

Significant debate remains about the use of awards programs to combat medical errors. While some argue that to highlight error reduction is to acknowledge publicly that errors exist, we do not believe this argument holds much value. Whether the industry likes it or not, the public is aware that such errors exist. The IOM report, consumer groups, and even government agencies provide guidance to patients on how to prevent medical errors. The Agency for Healthcare Research and Quality (2000) in Washington, D.C., produces an online guidebook for patients entitled *20 Tips to Prevent Medical Errors*. This and other awareness-building efforts will only accelerate and negate arguments against recognition.

Whether to compensate, however, is entirely another matter. During the heart of the quality movement in healthcare, a frequently asked question was whether quality teams should be paid for accomplishments. Deming was adamantly opposed to financial recognition, whereas Juran favored compensation under the right circumstances, and their followers have not come to terms with this issue, nor has a successful, long-term solution been discovered.

Toyota's suggestion system, which is much more focused and robust than any U.S. healthcare organization's we have observed, is one exception. They compensate, on average, $1,400 per person per year, when an economic benefit per person tops $37,000 (Yasuda 1991). Toyota's system has proven effective for them. Over half of Toyota subsidiaries enjoy participation rates above 90 percent, compared to the average U.S. company at 8 percent participation. There is some evidence that short-term programs can be very effective in healthcare. The VA established a Patient Safety Awards program in which up to $5,000 could be received for a major innovation replicable across the entire VA system (Kizer 2000).

State the Intent of the Initiative in Terms of the Organization's Mission, Vision, and Values

It probably goes without saying, but it is important to provide a link between any aggressive medication error reduction activity and the organization's mission, vision, and values. As suggested earlier, Reinertsen has declared that it is, in fact, CareGroup's vision to become the safest place in the world to receive medications. There is no doubt within the organization, from the board down to all the staff, that medication safety is what CareGroup is all about. Ken Kizer, M.D., architect of the successful VA efforts, believes that one of the reasons for the VA's accomplishments is that patient safety became a leadership priority from the beginning (Kizer 2000). Further, to be optimally effective, these activities should be incorporated into the organization's quality improvement plan, committee charters, or other appropriate tactical plans to ensure alignment of effort and to avoid duplication and counterproductive projects. One organization we visited recently had three major committees—medical staff, quality department, and patient care department—addressing medication error reduction, all seemingly competing to control this critical strategy. Some projects were, in fact, suboptimizing and negating the work of other committees.

Estimate the Resources Required

Although error reduction need not place a financial burden on the organization, underresourcing can become a major impediment. Several resource commitments become paramount in the course of mobilizing for the strategy.

The assurance of an adequate budget for benchmarking and research should be acknowledged up front. In addition, executive diligence, time, and attention is a prerequisite to success; executives should periodically scan their calendars in advance to ensure that no competing strategies will prevent their active involvement.

Moreover, the time required by managers, process owners, quality improvement (QI) staff, and analyst staff should be considered. Any aggressive initiative of this type is not something to pile on busy managers; if the managers are already at capacity for projects, examine the projects and time lines to determine which ones might be postponed and reassigned to other managers and quality staff. A rule-of-thumb estimate is that to implement one process change per month will require approximately two to four hours per month, or about 3 to 7 percent of the manager's work week. Embarking on any initiative without consideration of the time required, in advance, will bottleneck progress to the point of failure, particularly if an aggressive goal, such as a 25 percent reduction in 12 months, is established.

An effective technique to free up manager time is to conduct a breakout session at the medication error kickoff meeting to anticipate barriers to achieving the stretch goal of, say, 25 percent error reduction or implementing one process change per month. As potential barriers are raised, subsequent breakout groups are assigned the top ones to resolve. Typically, the number one barrier is lack of time. The breakout group trying to resolve this time barrier might propose, for example, reducing other meeting requirements for managers, delegating certain manager tasks to others, or even eliminating certain meetings and tasks.

Finally, a contingency plan should be established for freeing up capital to deploy idealized design change concepts. Technology—from information technology to robotics and diagnostic and therapeutic device upgrades—will play a significant role in achieving heroic gains in error reduction. Assessing capital availability over the next three years is an important mobilization task.

Deploy a Communication Plan

One task to be completed early (and often) is the development of a communication plan tailored to the needs of various constituency groups—boards, medical staff, referring physicians, managers, employees, and the community at large. Communications specialists typically advise that those closest to the initiative should feel that communications have been overdone. The success of the initiative will depend on the almost-constant repetition of goals and the organization's progress toward achieving them.

Redesign the Infrastructure for Speed

A critical feature of the 100-Day Plan management method is speed. Creative idea teams are chartered, measured, and held accountable for implementing one improvement every 30 days. These cycles are referred to as "ramps" (discussed in detail in the implementation step later in this chapter). Therefore, everything that follows is rooted in the 100-Day Plan design feature mandating speed of deployment. In fact, of all the features of this method, if only one could be sustained, it would be speed, which far outdistances all other success factors.

As the IHI Breakthrough Series mantra intones, "What can you do by next Tuesday?" Yet, as strong as the Breakthrough Series performance has been, approximately 25 percent of its participants are nonstarters. After several interviews with participants in their very successful "Reducing Adverse Drug Events" collaboratives, infrastructure emerged as a consistent theme (Leape et al. 1998). The following tasks establish an infrastructure capable of supporting and driving rapid implementation during the implementation step.

Charter the Creative Idea Committee

The creative idea committee is chaired by the executive change agent. Although it might go without saying, to ensure overall success, the CEO must fully empower the creative idea committee to make decisions for the system regarding capital, process changes, policy changes, and so on. Therefore, membership should come from the highest levels of the organization, including senior executives from operations, finance, medical staff affairs, patient care, quality improvement, and human resources. The creative idea committee meets monthly to review progress, appoint creative idea team leaders and members, and receive each creative idea team's initial deployment plan and subsequent monthly updates.

In the VA approach, a patient center was chartered that included an oversight committee, functioning as a creative idea committee, and also included an error event registry and feedback process as well as a lessons-learned process (Kizer 2000). Functioning in much the same way, at CareGroup's monthly meetings each executive shares a story of an adverse drug event. Reinertsen (2000) believes that, in addition to heightened awareness, the activity has had a strong effect on building a collaborative environment.

Frequently, executives and staff end up on committees of this type by default. In many cases, the mind-set appears to be that everyone with any possible connection to any potential solution is tapped to serve. The ideal selection method is first to determine critical criteria and the executive-level support required to drive medication error reduction and then to appoint logical individuals. Those with moderate or slight influence on potential solutions, such as the CFO or CIO, should be appointed as ex officio or ad hoc members (which is generally appreciated because of their other, pressing priorities). However, it is usually better to follow an inclusive rather than an exclusive approach and welcome any executive with a passion for this initiative.

Appoint a Facilitator to Manage the Creative Idea Committee

In addition to an executive change agent, every successful initiative seems to have a facilitator, someone who is accountable on a day-to-day basis for ensuring that projects, time lines, measures, and managers stay focused. The characteristics of an effective facilitator for medication error reduction are the same as those for quality improvement teams. The facilitator should possess exceptionally strong project management skills and the ability to learn new concepts quickly, followed closely by communication and meeting planning capabilities. Analytic abilities round out the list. Much less important is medication management, nursing care, or clinical knowledge, although such knowledge would be a plus.

It has been our experience that inside staff seem to wear out their welcome from time to time and outside facilitator support accelerates the effort. Sharing a facilitator among IDN campuses can overcome this obstacle, as would the engagement of an outside consultant to support efforts for the first 6 to 12 months. In the absence of an outside resource, the organization should place its strongest facilitator on this initiative and not simply someone who has the available time. Generally, our recommendation is to identify the strongest facilitator in the organization and then reassign his or her current projects to other facilitators.

Determine the Core Processes with the Greatest Incidences of Error

Much more is known about the etiology and effective countermeasures for medication error prevention and mitigation than other process categories, except perhaps nosocomial infections. There are a number of different ways to approach this issue. Errors can be looked at by cost, occurrence, source, and process and functional area, with even further distillation. Organizations can examine only the subset of total medication errors that produce compensable events, potentially compensable events, adverse drug events, preventable adverse reactions, near misses, or total medication errors.

We support addressing the broadest possible view of medication errors, prioritizing initial interventions at those areas causing the most harm in terms of human suffering and avoidable costs for society, and then working down the list until significant progress toward six sigma levels is achieved. If, in fact, patient safety and medical error reduction is to be a significant part of an organization's vision and strategy, it must be multiyear and all encompassing.

The current body of knowledge permits organizations to approach reduction from a number of angles. From a cost perspective, the greatest source of errors, including medication-related errors and other errors, is surgical and anesthesia events (Advisory Board Company 1999), which comprise, on average, 44 percent of the cost of total medical errors, with an undisclosed percentage of those costs from medication errors. Nosocomial infections cost 20 percent of the total, and adverse drug events 14 percent. However, by occurrence, Leape et al. (1991) has shown that 19 percent of total errors are medication related, followed by wound infections at 14 percent. Work by David Bates at the Brigham and Women's Hospital points to 30 percent of medication error occurrences from anesthesia, 24 percent from antibiotic use, and 8 percent from sedatives (Bates et al. 1997).

Michael Cohen (1998) at the Institute for Safe Medication Practices (ISMP) found that errors tend to occur in the following types of drugs:

Insulin	11.0 %
Heparin	8.9 %
Opiate	8.0 %
Allergic	4.3 %
Potassium related	3.3 %
PCA pump related	2.3 %

Some hints about how to approach medication error reduction also can be derived by examining the process causes of errors and process failures as Leape has done (Leape et al. 1991):

Causes of Error

Lack of drug knowledge	22 %
Lack of patient information	14 %
Policy/Procedure violation	10 %
Slips	9 %
Transcription	9 %

Process Failures

Drug knowledge dissemination	29 %
Dose and patient identity checking	12 %
Patient info availability	11 %
Order transcription	9 %
Allergy alerts	7 %

Finally, and perhaps most revealing, Leape et al. (1991) examined the sources of medication errors and the percentage of errors intercepted (near misses):

	Source	Interceptions
M.D. prescribing	39 %	48 %
Nurse administering	38 %	2 %
Transcription	12 %	33 %
Pharmacist	11 %	34 %

Although it might be beneficial to construct similar research within your organization, we do not suggest postponing deployment of known process interventions such as those proposed in chapter 5. Rather, we suggest beginning to improve now while collecting data for the next project, asking which processes have the greatest adverse drug events and medication errors nested within them.

Viewed in these ways, the processes with the greatest potential and the least mitigation are administration and physician prescribing. A later discussion of creative idea teams and potential interventions will show that the role for pharmacists and health information/medical records staff should

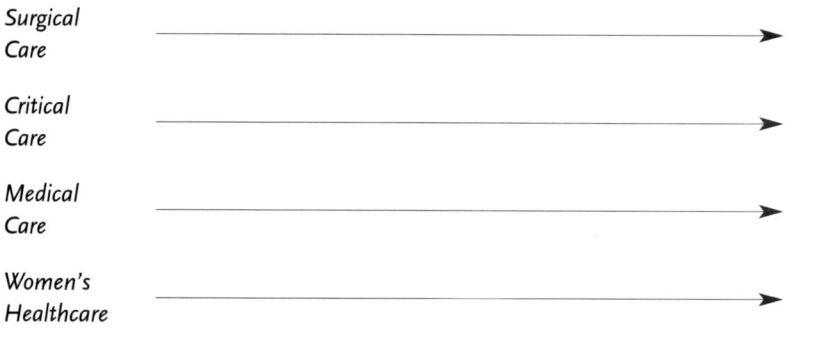

FIGURE 4.4. HIGH-LEVEL MEDICATION MANAGEMENT FLOWCHART

be deployed on prescribing and administration creative idea teams because they are part of the extended core processes involved.

Construct High-Level Flowcharts to Scope the Initiative and Identify Logical Process Owners

We can construct a two-way, high-level flowchart and determine critical process owners for both subprocesses and functional areas, as suggested in Figure 4.4.

Identify Influencers of Each Core Process

After we have some sense of the process interplay, both horizontally and vertically, we can ensure that the appropriate process owners and influencers are engaged. It is not necessary to identify and appoint different individuals from a subprocess. For example, one pharmacist and one health information management/medical records person might be appointed to interface with each team.

Charter Creative Idea Teams

After determining processes and their owners and influencers, we can designate creative idea team membership. We tend to support attacking med-

FIGURE 4.5.   CREATIVE IDEA TEAM STRUCTURE

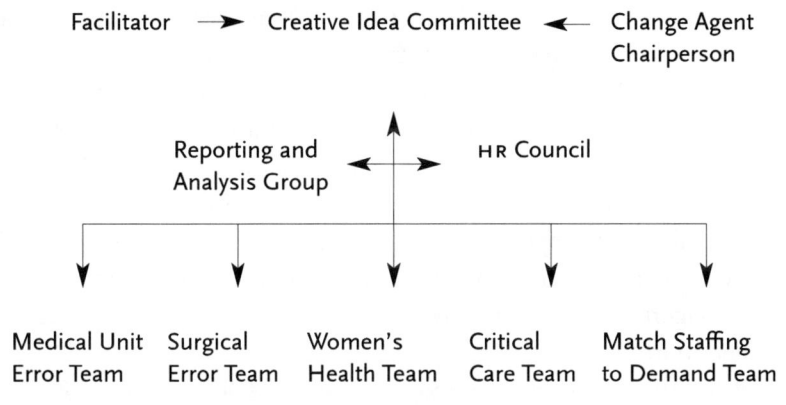

Reprinted with permission. *Chip Caldwell & Associates, LLC.*

ical errors broadly and medication errors, in particular, by process, rather than by error type. Further, we suggest that the work be done by a logical team composed of individuals who work within that process, meaning within the same functional area or department. In other words, we encourage the formation, for example, of the critical care team, the surgical team, and the orthopedic unit team, rather than forming separate teams for nosocomial infections, antibiotic use, analgesics use, etc.

The reasons for this bias are twofold. First, process owners and functional areas have a tendency to work as teams, as colleagues around all subprocesses and extensions of core processes within the functional area. The same nursing personnel, pharmacists, respiratory therapists, physicians, and support staff frequent the critical care unit, visit the orthopedic floor, and interact in each surgical department. By organizing the medical error initiative broadly, and the medication error initiative specifically, by functional area or department, we are capitalizing on existing relationships. Further, as we attack other priorities, such as antibiotic use or nosocomial infections, we are building on successes from the previous initiative, rather than having to create a new team. An effective team must transition through four stages—"form, storm, norm, then perform"— to emerge as a fully optimized work group. This melding of interpersonal characteristics requires work, patience, effort, and, most scarce, time.

Further, we suggest organizing creative idea teams as shown in Figure 4.5.

In addition to the process-focused creative idea teams, you will note other teams. The reporting and analysis group is charged with establishing, maintaining, and improving the error-reporting processes, including the analysis and deployment of technology to capture adverse drug events and medication errors. Perhaps the toughest job in the beginning, as reported by organizations with advanced medication error reduction teams, is to actually detect errors. Both the VA and SSM Health Care reported that, initially, errors increased as they innovated detection processes and began the process of eliminating the fear of reporting (Spreadbury 2000; Kizer 2000). This task falls to the reporting and analysis group. It is also this group's job to manage the improvement process, collect monthly improvement reports from managers, and construct trend graphs and other reports for the creative idea committee.

The match staffing to demand team and the human resources (HR) council are discussed in chapter 6, but, briefly, their roles are to convert the time saved from error reduction into productivity gains. The match staffing to demand team applies change concepts that convert time saved into redesigned staffing processes, and the HR council manages the organization's position control log of authorized positions. Although these teams operate in tandem with medication error reduction teams, their role is much broader, encompassing many advanced techniques to redeploy staff to areas where appropriate demand exists.

After determining which creative idea teams to charter, the next task is to determine team membership and appoint an influencer to head each team. (Refer to chapter 7, section II, step 1, for an exercise on appointing appropriate staff to these teams.)

Finally, each creative idea team should be given a clear goal with a measurable intention. This goal, established early in the deployment of the medication error reduction strategy, prevents any misunderstanding or loss of focus as the creative idea teams charter projects, coordinate with other teams, make recommendations regarding technology deployment, and undertake other tasks to achieve the measurable goal.

Redesign All Decision Processes for Speed

One critical factor that is very often, but not always, overlooked is speed of deployment. In a study of characteristics of high-performance companies in the microcomputer and biotechnology industries, Paul Stepanovich found that speedy decision making was instrumental in achieving high performance (Stepanovich and Uhrig 1999). In relating those characteristics required of healthcare organizations in high-velocity environments, five factors emerged:

1. Fast-paced companies analyze and react to data quickly and do not wait until the perfect data set is available or automated.
2. Multiple solutions are considered simultaneously versus preconceived solutions or only two or three alternatives.
3. Independent, knowledgeable thinkers, sometimes from outside the process, are used to gather multiple viewpoints before taking action.
4. A consensus, or "I can live with that," approach to decision making is used, rather than waiting until all agree on only one solution.
5. A disciplined implementation process, such as the 100-Day Plan, is used that encompasses multiple affected departments and functions.

Decision-making processes are just like other processes, such as medication administration or clinical paths. They follow a logical, sequential order until resolution occurs. Often, however, management processes such as decision making or staffing are not thought of as processes and do not enjoy the same level of improvement rigor that nonmanagement processes do. However, these processes often have a more substantial effect on improvement than do most others.

During a 1999 quality-based cost reduction analysis for a large midwestern IDN and its wholly owned HMO, our consulting team at Chip Caldwell & Associates constructed a cash flow analysis based on speed of deployment. The analysis showed that to achieve the IDN's multimillion-dollar target, two dependent variables were vital to consider—speed of implementation, and magnitude of each individual change. It was pointed out that, for all ten teams, if they could implement each idea in 30 days or less, each change only required an effect of $83,000. However, if decisions required 90 days to implement, individual changes must achieve an effect of $250,000 each. As it turned out, the organization required much longer than even 90 days, and for the first time in its history, the IDN suffered a negative margin.

Another example from a New England academic center further illustrates the importance of speed of decision making. In attempting to influence antibiotic improvements, the clinical chiefs acknowledged that for a formulary change to be completed, the section must make the recommendation to the department, which then forwarded it to a pharmacy and therapeutics committee, which then recommended the change to an executive committee. Under a certain scenario, it might require as long as six months to formalize a change that those closest to the care process—the surgeons themselves—agree needs to be made. The reason, by the way, for the formalized structure was stated to be the Joint Commission on Accreditation of Healthcare Organization (JCAHO) criteria. After review by the quality department, it was determined that the JCAHO criteria did not mandate a specific routing but, instead, mandated only that certain critical committees review each change. Therefore, the medical center was able to alter its policy so that each section was empowered to make critical changes and their changes still routed through the various committees, not for approval but, rather, for ratification. Any upstream committee could reverse the change for quality reasons, but the section could immediately implement it. In this case, the speed of decision making was reduced from six months to zero.

To uncover bottlenecks in the decision-making process, a simple exercise has proved effective. During the kickoff of the medication error reduction initiative, or at some other convenient gathering, assemble creative idea team members for a three-hour decision-making process redesign session. Divide members into different groups and ask them to brainstorm and nominally group barriers to speedy decisions. Their list will most likely be complete and comprehensive. After report-outs by each group, select the top four or five barriers and reassign team members to new groups designated to brainstorm creative solutions to each identified barrier. Again, conduct report-outs. Upon conclusion, the reporting and analysis group should construct leading barriers and potential solutions for the creative idea committee to implement.

Train Staff in the Core Competencies Required to Implement Idealized Design Change Concepts

Most executives underestimate the importance of ongoing training, particularly in this environment of rapid change. Executives seem to have the sense that managers in today's cost-driven (and now safety-focused) environment possess all the management skills required to drive out non-value-added cost and error-prone process steps. Not long ago, a respected comparative data executive stated at a national conference, "If you just give comparative data to good managers, they will know what to do." That may have been true five years ago, but it is no longer accurate. Reflect on the initiatives within your own organization. How many cost reduction programs have come and gone? How many improvement activities have been completed?

During a $48 million cost reduction project in a midsized Florida IDN, our consulting team was assisting a manager in constructing his plan to remove a significant number of full-time employees from his department. Many senior executives have not been exposed to the ramifications and implications of aggressive cost reduction initiatives at the department manager level. Moreover, most managers will not confide in the CEO or senior executives when they have no solutions because of either fear or pride, or both. Regardless, it was apparent that this department manager had no clue. This particular organization, because of intense competition with a rival health system, had already achieved top-quartile performance in cost and productivity. Therefore, many of the managers, particularly this one, had implemented most of the ideas known to them. To complicate matters, the physicians practicing in this department had informed him in no uncertain terms that they would not collaborate in further cost reduction initiatives. As a result, this manager, normally very composed, articulate, and confident, and recognized by his peers as a leader among them, told us that he had no idea what to do and knew that he would be fired. He was simply terrified and mostly immobilized.

We do not believe that he is alone among his colleagues nationally. Many managers have simply implemented the ideas known to them. More troublesome, the rate of speed necessary to achieve organizational survival has increased dramatically. Managers today have been placed in management situations for which they have not been prepared and, in most cases, are not being given the training and tools needed to succeed.

To accomplish any heroic goal, particularly medication error reduction, organizations must reexamine the investments they are making in training, coaching and mentoring, and education.

During the American College of Healthcare Executives's quality-based cost reduction course, Jim Brexler and Chip Caldwell conducted an exercise probing for skills that are critical for managers who hope to succeed in the future. The following list summarizes those skills believed critical by CEOS and executives who contributed to the course over the past two years:

- Comparative data interpretation.
- Basic analytic statistical methods (trended data streams) and interpretation (not production) of statistical process control charts.
- Process benchmarking phone interview preparation, conduct, analysis, and execution. Many managers presume that simply knowing whom to call is adequate, but many hours of effort are often suboptimized because the wrong questions were posed to the interviewee. Process benchmarking requires a certain understanding of which process-focused questions to ask and how to probe for information that can be acted on.
- Applied research. Tools such as nih.gov, MedLine, Google.com, and other Internet search engines abound. The ability to rapidly identify materials that are mission critical to rapid project deployment requires an investment in training and case-study development.
- Idealized design and change concepts (as will be discussed in chapter 5).
- Creativity to incorporate change concepts into the organization's unique processes and culture.

- Driving change and management of resistance.
- Project management.
- Quality control and service recovery.

Establish Measurement and Tracking Processes

Another vital component of the 100-Day Plan is the establishment of measurement and tracking processes. The final task in generating organizational will is to establish a measurement set, or refine it, if one already exists. There are three types of measurement sets that organizations can and should deploy:

- strategic measures;
- project measures; and
- quality control measures.

At this point, we are constructing a long-term strategic measurement set, not project measurement or quality control measures. Therefore, our purposes are different than they are for short-term project measurement. Generally, organizations try to place too many variables in the strategic measurement set and get lost in the details. We suggest creating some measurement deployment guidelines to ensure consistency across the organization and that all managers are using measurement effectively. The following objectives will help you to:

- capture only those measures that will be acted on.
- link activity with results. Some measures of outcome and some measures of the number of projects completed and improvements made are more important than others. For strategic measures, or balanced scorecard purposes, it is more important to measure execution and implementation on a monthly basis and then measure outcomes on either a monthly or quarterly basis.
- view medical error rates, in general, and medication error rates, in particular, along with productivity measures for the underlying processes. In other words, to measure the medication cost per discharge, patient care hours per patient day, and pharmacy department cost per prescription side by side with error rates.
- measure as little as possible to ensure that the strategic goal is achieved and to monitor, at a high level, those process characteristics critical to our mission and vision. Therefore, the measurement should have an actual data stream, a minimum goal or "panic" point, and a stretch goal.

- measure only as often as action will be taken on the measurement in the event a performance threshold is missed. Why measure weekly or monthly if the intention is to only act quarterly?
- see as much information as possible on one page. That is why the balanced scorecard, or spider diagram, is a preferred measurement tool for strategic measures.
- see the effects of process variation because of staff, seasonal, and other variables. Trended data are preferable to static data forms—run charts and statistical process control (SPC) charts are preferable to bar charts.
- cascade measurement logically from the CEO level through the VP level and the process level to the manager level, keeping the number of measures as low as possible. Many CEO strategic measurement sets include measures that belong on the CFO or chief medical officer set. For example, the CEO set should include only the one or two highest-level financial measures, such as "operating expenses as a percent of net revenue." The CFO set should include the two or three subprocess measures driving the CEO measure. For example, to support the CEO measure above, the CFO might measure "FTES per adjusted occupied bed" and "supply expense as a percent of total operating expense."

Several key considerations are important in deploying a measurement set:

- What do executives and managers need to measure to achieve the goal?
- Why should we measure this process characteristic? What will it tell us that we do not already know? At the start of measurement set creation, we have found that the organization lays out every possible measurement, covering every conceivable contingency. Measurement is not the enjoyable part of improvement so it should be kept to the minimum that will be used.
- Who will act on this information if it is provided? If the answer is that a senior executive or manager will act quickly and decisively, it passes the critical test. If the answer is vague, drop the measure and consider it for a project measure (usually temporary) or quality control measure (usually measured infrequently or at the staff level).
- How often will we take action should a variation from threshold occur? If action would be taken immediately, the measurement should be considered for daily, weekly, or monthly plotting. If we would only act on the variation quarterly, a quarterly measurement should suffice. Generally speaking, most executive measures are better suited for quarterly or monthly measurement.

- How can we best learn from this information, or what is the best format to use? Should we trend the data or look at them in isolation from other data streams? As a general rule, trended information provides more information than static information, that is, run charts of small sample sizes as opposed to bar charts.
- What is the source of the data? If automated, such as patient care hours per patient day or pharmacy cost per prescription, how often are the data available? For data requiring manual collection processes, a host of complicating factors is present. How often? Who collects? Who analyzes? How large a sample is necessary? Ask the quality department or others charged with the analysis function to provide a brief training session using three exceptional resources: *How to Use Control Charts for Healthcare* (Kelly 1999); *The Improvement Guide* (Langley et al. 1996); and *Reducing Adverse Drug Events* (Leape et al. 1998).
- How many data points should we collect and plot? The answer to this question is different for strategic measurement sets than for projects and quality control. For strategic measures, most measures are automated, particularly financial data. For those that are not, small sample sizes serve our purposes very well. Because we are trending data over time, we take less risk that an inappropriate action, or tampering, will occur. While this question usually raises much debate, the first question to ask is, "How much data exist now from which you make critical judgments?" The answer is most often little or none, so going from one extreme to the other is usually not the best advice.
- For measures that are available only infrequently, should we supplement the data? For example, patient satisfaction data are usually provided semiannually, but we often wish to spot trends well before six to nine months have passed. Therefore, we should determine whether an adequate proxy exists that can be sampled more frequently. In this case, complaints supplement nicely. The same is true for medication error rates. At present, few organizations measure medication error rates or surgical error rates. One fear is that organizations will apply more resources than are required to medication error rate measurement and fewer than are required to measure the execution of process changes.

Taking all these factors into account, three measurement tools aid the creative idea committee in its work:

1. the 100-Day milestones tracking chart;
2. the organization's balanced scorecard; and
3. an effective cascade of measures.

FIGURE 4.6. 100-DAY MILESTONES TRACKING

FY00 ACTUAL

MM	Stretch	Actual
Customer satisfaction	83%	Hit stretch
Contribution margin	160% of budget	Hit stretch
Revenue	130% of budget	Below target
Penetrate new markets	10 new market segments	Hit stretch
Reduce medication errors 25%	30%	Hit target

FY01 YTD STATUS

MM	Stretch	Status
Customer satisfaction	83%	Above stretch
Contribution margin	105% budget	Below target
Revenue	105% budget	Below target
70% managers achieve "4" or "5"	80%	Above stretch
Medication errors 25%	30%	Above stretch

FY01 1Q STATUS (2nd 100-day period)

MM	Stretch
Customer satisfaction	NM
Contribution margin	105%
Gross revenue	105%
30% managers at "4" or "5"	35%
Medication errors 25%	30%

PROPOSED FY02 GOALS

MM	Stretch
Customer satisfaction	83%
Contribution margin	105% of budget
Gross revenue	105% of budget
70% managers at "4" or "5"	80%
Surgical errors	30%

Source: Larry Abramson, Premier, Inc. 2/2000
Reprinted with permission. Chip Caldwell & Associates, LLC.

First, the 100-Day milestones tracking chart illustrated in Figure 4.6 provides a view of the preceding fiscal year, goal accomplishment for the next fiscal year, and the current year-to-date and current quarter. This tool provides critical measurement of both outcomes and activity, or results matched to execution.

The 100-Day milestones tracking chart measurement tool supplements the second measurement tool, an organization's balanced scorecard (see Figure 4.7). A typical scorecard contains 8 to 20 measures, along with each measure's panic value, stretch value, and current value (Caldwell 1995). Detailed discussion regarding the establishment and management of a balanced scorecard process is beyond the scope of this manuscript. For information on how to set up an organizationwide scorecard, refer to *Mentoring Strategic Change in Health Care* (Caldwell 1995).

The third measurement tool is a cascade of measures that begins with the CEO-level measures, through the VP level, all the way down through the organization to the department manager level. The measure scheme is logically linked so that efforts to improve CEO-level measures can be tracked throughout the organization. This concept can be seen as creating a line of sight from the CEO to the department manager. As an example, if one of the CEO measures is patient satisfaction percent, then the chief patient care executive measure linked to this measure might be the patient satisfaction question, "Did nursing staff respond to your requests in a timely manner?" Then each nursing unit manager would track "Minutes to answer call lights" as a key performance indicator.

Following is an example of an effective cascade of measures for medication error reduction:

Measure	Level	Frequency
Medication errors per adjusted discharge	CEO balanced scorecard, 100-day milestones tracking, creative idea committee balanced scorecard, and medication errors team	Quarterly
Percent of managers achieving a "4" or "5" on the monthly manager activity results report card	CEO balanced scorecard, 100-day milestones tracking, creative idea committee monthly medication error team activity results report card	Monthly
Operating cost per adjusted discharge	CEO balanced scorecard, 100-day milestones tracking	Monthly
FTES per adjusted occupied bed	CFO balanced scorecard or trend graphs, match staffing to demand team	Monthly
Direct staff to total staff ratio	CFO balanced scorecard or trend graphs, match staffing to demand team	Monthly

Adverse events per discharge	Medication errors team	Quarterly*
Prescribing errors per prescription	Medication errors team	Quarterly*
Ordering errors per prescription	Medication errors team	Quarterly*
Drug preparation errors per prescription	Medication errors team	Quarterly*
Administration error per prescription	Medication errors team	Quarterly*
Medication process cost per discharge (including staff cost) (or the proxy pharmacy department total cost and all patient care units total cost)	Medication errors team	Quarterly*
Patient care hours per patient day	VP, patient care/chief nursing officer balanced scorecard, match staffing to demand team	Monthly
Indirect RN staff to total RN staff ratio	VP, patient care/chief nursing officer balanced scorecard, match staffing to demand team	Monthly
Pharmacy cost per prescription	Pharmacy director	Monthly

*(or monthly if the focus of an active project)

These 14 measures shown in the table form the strategic measurement set for the medication error reduction initiative. As the organization deploys initiatives to tackle surgical errors, critical care errors, and patient care errors, a similar deployment can be used. It is important to keep in mind that the CEO-level measurement set should be the highest level and should contain only one measure.

Along with the strategic measures above, project-specific measures also will be deployed on a temporary basis as long as that project is active. For example, the medication errors team might initially tackle improvements in the process to identify known and unknown patient allergies. For this project-level measurement, the team may wish to track allergy-related medication errors (adverse drug events, other medication errors, and near misses).

Finally, to more strongly link activity to results, the monthly medication error team activity results report card charts the degree of results from the

FIGURE 4.7. SAFETY-FOCUSED BALANCED SCORECARD

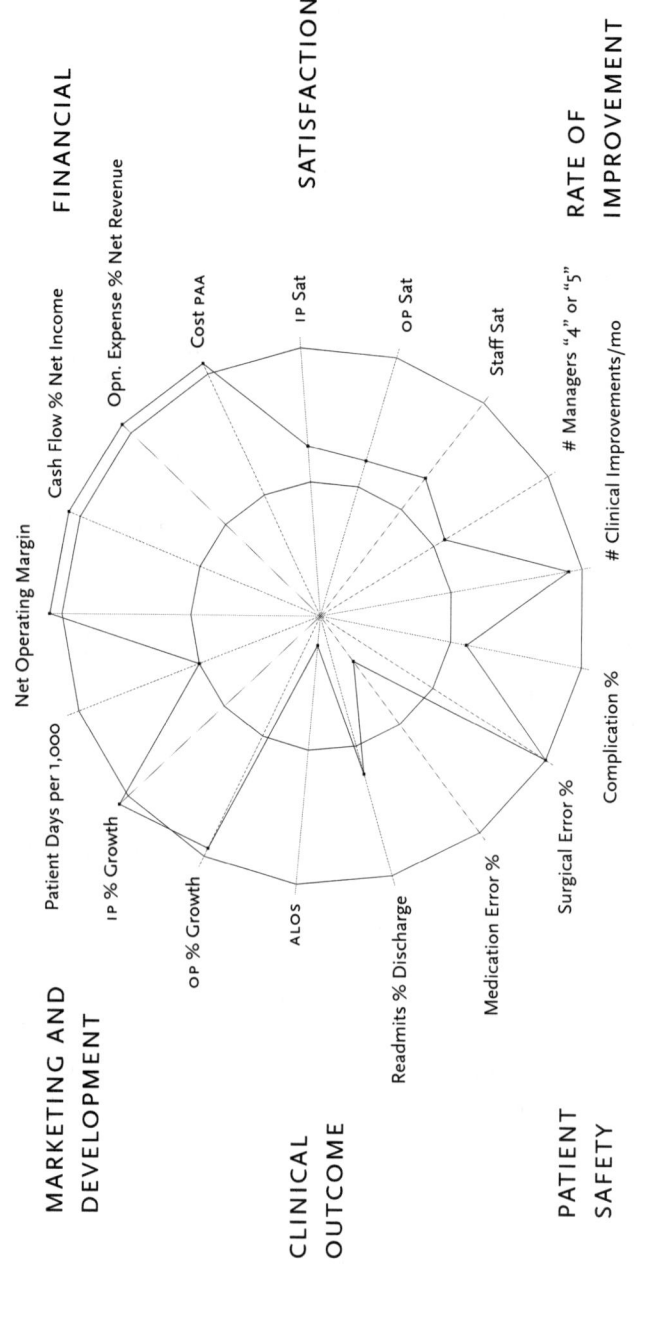

Reprinted with permission. Chip Caldwell & Associates, LLC.

FIGURE 4.8. MONTHLY MEDICATION ERROR TEAM ACTIVITY
RESULTS REPORT CARD

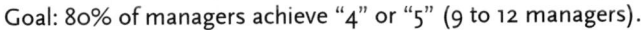

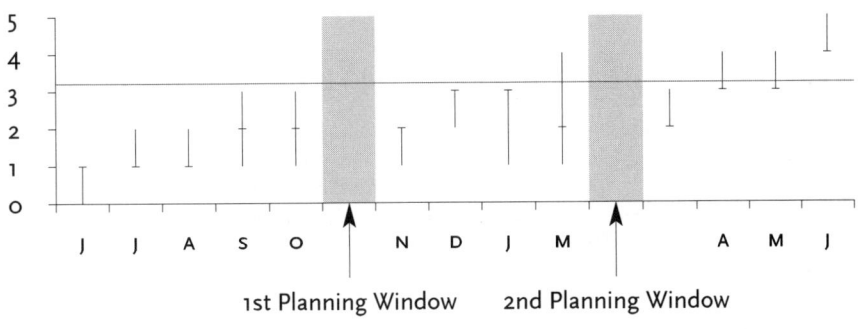

exertion of manager execution. It also tracks, in our opinion, the most important strategic factor—speed of implementation. As is discussed later in the idealized design implementation step, each month managers score the effect of their activity implemented during the month. The average and range of these scores is a critical CEO and creative idea committee measure, found in both the 100-day milestones tracking form and the balanced scorecard. The scoring, adapted from the successful IHI Breakthrough Series model, links manager activity to results (Leape et al. 1998). The importance of strategically linking activity with results or, conversely, outcomes to managerial effort, cannot be understated. Deploying the rigor at the CEO, executive, and creative idea committee levels of matching the projects undertaken by the organization and management changes made by individual managers ensures that all are focused on the same objectives. Measuring the relationship between organizational effort and results can be a very powerful tool. Figure 4.8 provides a sample of this measurement.

Leveraging Step 1 for Success

All successful management systems, including the 100-Day Plan, face barriers and obstacles that suboptimize effective deployment. Some of the leverage factors to manage include:

- loss of senior leader resolve or active engagement;
- false starts;
- "analysis paralysis";
- too many priorities;
- waiting for the perfect solution or perfect measurement set; and
- use of the 100-day milestones tracking form and the monthly medication error team activity results report card.

STEP 2. CONDUCT A COMPARATIVE DATA AND GAP ANALYSIS

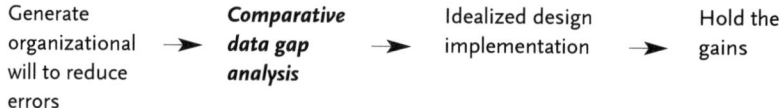

Generate organizational will to reduce errors → **Comparative data gap analysis** → Idealized design implementation → Hold the gains

Whereas the effect of step 1 promises an infrastructure and measurement process capable of driving and sustaining rapid medication error reduction (the foundation, if you will), the outcome of step 2 provides the direction. If we think of the organizational will process as preparing for the trip, the comparative data and gap analysis provide the road map to get there. It contains the compass, mapping tools, and all the necessary aids to determine what needs to be done to arrive at our destination. The output of step 2 is the publication of three-year objectives and one-year goals for the medication error team following the processes described below.

Set Targets Using Comparative Data

The first activity in this second step of the 100-Day Plan management method is to set targets for the medication error team and the match staffing to demand team.

Medication Error Team Goals

Using the strategic measures relative to the medication error team constructed in step 1, the team examines the organization's performance for adverse drug events per discharge and medication errors per discharge. This, of course, produces two complexities that consistently arose during our interviews: the inherent error rate from self-reporting, and the shortage of comparative data not subject to peer review.

As discussed earlier, the available benchmark data suggest a range of options. Quite frankly, the comparison to other organizations for any error classification, including adverse drug events and medication errors, helps very little and perhaps even harms the degree of urgency that comparative analysis usually imparts. The industry requires heroic improvement levels, perhaps higher than the tenfold threshold set by Tom Nolan and the IHI. Therefore, the benchmark chosen is only helpful to console the organization that others have just as high a mountain to climb as it does, but is not very helpful in setting a world-class standard to achieve. We suggest investing little time constructing benchmarking research unless you believe a world-class standard exists in the healthcare industry. For urgency's sake, we encourage adoption of Bates's benchmark of 1.8 percent adverse drug events per discharge and Leape's 10 percent medication errors per discharge.

A caveat about setting goals based on comparative information, shared with us by Ken Sands, M.D., and Saul Weingart, M.D., of CareGroup's Beth Israel Deaconess Medical Center, is worth noting at this point. Because medical error data, in general, and medication errors, in particular, require at least some form of manual collection (if not 100 percent), avoid waiting to implement process changes until a baseline is determined. Success will depend on achieving a very low error rate; this will be accomplished through many large and small process changes and speed is not aided by waiting to construct a baseline that will not be enlightening. The effect of relying on manual processes is a high variation in error reporting, unit to unit, entity to entity, health system to health system; and this is further complicated by the unknown, and thus questionable, value of external benchmark data not subjected to the rigor of studies published in peer-reviewed journals. The most effective benchmark will likely be your own past. Mayo Luther Midelfort Health System found self-benchmarking more valuable than external comparison. Bill Rupp, M.D., president and CEO, remarked, "But to me, [achieving the national average] means one out of ten of our patients isn't getting the appropriate care, and that doesn't sound so good. We want to raise the standards tenfold or more, and benchmarking against others isn't really helpful in doing that" (National Health Information 2000).

The field of medical errors presents an interesting dilemma because, unlike clinical and operations processes, no universal data set exists for medical errors or, for that matter, any single category of medical errors, such as medication errors. If you have seen one medical errors measurement system, you have seen one measurement system. Even in integrated delivery systems that have deployed one common software tool for the retrospective collection of medical errors, the definition of an error often differs from one site to the next. This lack of a consistent, standardized model in the industry presents an interesting, but not insurmountable, difficulty. The following steps might prove useful.

1. Start with existing comparative data sources for hints and proxies for the presence of errors. Using clinical test–level detail, determine variances from top-quartile performance in drug utilization and cost, surgery utilization and cost, and other potential proxies for the presence of overuse and misuse errors. Then, examine operations' comparative databases for productivity variances that often signify labor costs incurred because of overuse or misuse errors. Although beyond the scope of this book, the evolving field of cost comparative data collection and analysis has solved many of the legitimate concerns about comparability of costs across institutional and regional lines. Case-mix adjustment, regional adjustment, and peer group selection go a long way toward creating an "apples and apples" analysis. However, one point worth noting is that many strategists carry their expectations too far. The purpose of comparative information is not to budget a particular clinical service line or department but, rather, to ensure that organizational effort is expended in the most effective processes and the relative magnitude of the opportunity is known. Comparative data have never been intended to meet the statistical rigor expected of clinical trials research or similar projects. Brent James, M.D., vice president of Intermountain Healthcare, and an internationally recognized expert in this area, states it best: "We are not looking for statistical significance, we are looking to assure we are directionally correct" (James 1999). In other words, the appropriate use of comparative data is to establish creative idea teams and allow them to prioritize their potential projects.

2. In the absence of comparative information, try to select processes with relatively high incidents of error and/or estimated quality recovery costs compared to other internal processes (for example, reports from the pharmacy system, supply chain, and risk management or quality management reports such as nosocomial infections and surgical wound infection analysis). Because we are trying to be directionally correct, not statistically significant, consider proxies for the presence of errors. Complaint logs, call logs to physicians by patient care staff, and other existing data may produce useful information with a little effort and creativity. An important consideration at this juncture is to move into comparative data analysis and move out of the process as quickly as possible. Every moment spent collecting data is one in which improvement work is not occurring. This is not to suggest proceeding without data necessary for planning or prioritizing but, rather, that "analysis paralysis" should be avoided. A helpful thought process is to ask, "How likely is it that additional data will change our priorities?"

3. Set three-year stretch objectives. Often during the review of the 100-Day Plan method, tasks critical to the overall success of the approach

have been pointed out. This is one of those critical tasks. As revealed in the analysis of GE's world dominance and factors driving IHI's unparalleled results, the deployment of stretch goals stands out. Recall the results of the first IHI Adverse Drug Event Breakthrough Series discussed previously. Most participants initially balked at the 12-month goal to reduce adverse drug events by 30 percent. Yet, of the 43 collaborators, 75 percent made "notable" progress, and 30 percent exceeded the 30 percent reduction goal (Leape et al. 1998). Objectives should be high-level ("reduce adverse drug events by 50 percent in three years") rather than process-specific ("increase the percentage of two-hour first-dose antibiotic administration on neurosciences units by 50 percent in three years"). The reason for this high-level approach, as is shown below, is that it is necessary to maintain a broad berth so that projects such as the antibiotic timing project above can be chartered at both the process and the department levels.

4. Set a one-year stretch goal using the same logic as that used in establishing three-year objectives. Our experience has shown that the last year is the most difficult. Therefore, consider allocating the three targets in disproportionate amounts, for example, allocating 50 percent of the goal in year one (allowing approximately three months to establish an acceptably stable error collection process), 50 percent of the remaining amount in year two, and the remainder in year three. For a 50 percent three-year stretch goal, therefore, achievement of the year one target would result in an overall reduction of 25 percent, leaving 12.5 percent each for years two and three.

Match Staffing to Demand Team Goals

A similar process is followed to set goals for the match staffing to demand team. As medical error teams, particularly the medication error team, reduce error, the result is saved staff time. It was the concept of recapturing lost productivity from defects and errors that revitalized the U.S. automobile industry in the 1980s and 1990s. Productivity rose tenfold, whereas defects declined a hundredfold.

Likewise in healthcare, it is important to recapture the time saved to productivity gains. However, rather than diverting to the review of six sigma concepts and the relationship between quality, patient safety, and productivity at this juncture, we have devoted chapter 6 "Knowledge Management Loop to Match Staffing to Demand" to a detailed discussion of this strategic imperative. Suffice it to acknowledge at this point that no quality or patient safety initiative is strategically complete without improvement processes to convert time saved from error reduction into staff productivity gains.

Two high-level goals can be recommended for the match staffing to demand team, as follows:

1. Recapture 70 percent of time saved by creative idea teams (medication error team, surgical error team, critical care error team, and patient care error team) into measurable productivity gains within 90 days of each project team implementation.
2. Achieve and maintain productivity per unit of service at the top-quartile level in 90 percent of departments within three years.

Of course, these goals can be raised depending on the current productivity performance of major departments in the IDN or organization. However, we do not recommend setting goals below top-quartile performance for any core process, function, diagnosis-related group (DRG), or department; rather, if the organization finds it is above the median, retain top quartile as the ultimate goal but increase the number of months to achieve it and set interim milestone goals to get there.

Consider some final examples about setting and achieving stretch goals for all creative idea teams under the creative idea committee, including the medication error and the match staffing to demand teams. As discussed in chapter 3, Jack Welch taught the field of management many critical lessons. One of these was that when faced with the impossible, the impossible is achieved. Conversely, when executives, managers, and teams reduce a truly stretch goal because they cannot at the moment determine the actions to achieve it, they tend to achieve what they set out to achieve. Welch compares this thought process to the annual budget-setting process. During the budgeting process, department managers invest significant time and energy to set a budget that is 120 percent achievable. The CFO and executives, on the other hand, without any underlying data to support their position, go into the annual budget cycle ready to increase each manager's original budget. Knowing this, the managers artificially set their budgets low so they can be heroes by raising their original projections (Welch 1996). Individuals and teams appear to get out of the box, engage in breakthrough thinking, and execute more flawlessly when faced with aggressive goals than they do when faced with moderate goals. The IHI Breakthrough Series mentioned earlier supports Welch's observations. The initial goal of 30 percent adverse drug event reduction was seen as insurmountable—yet, due to the stretch goal, over 30 percent exceeded it.

Another critical lesson revealed by Welch is that organizations using a stretch approach cannot use failure as a rationale for punitive action. Stretch goals that are set effectively will produce superlative results every single time, but stretch will not always be achieved. This is why the inner performance indicator of the balanced scorecard—the circle in the center of the spider diagram—is set at budget or minimally acceptable improvement. In turn, for strategic imperatives, stretch goal thresholds are designated as the outer circle and maintenance indicators are held at current or slightly higher performance.

Charter Projects Aligned to Targets

Now that three-year objectives and one-year goals have been established for the medication error and match staffing to demand teams, specific projects can be chartered. This can be done in six steps.

1. Assess the Magnitude of the Challenge

The process of project chartering begins by assessing the magnitude of the challenge. If true stretch goals were established, team members should be in some discomfort, visibly anxious about their ability to achieve the goals. A good sign would be if some team members were to express that achievement of these goals would mark a notable point in their professional careers.

The teams in the first and second sessions should envision the future state. Some team members will embrace this world-class state with vigor; others will be overcome with the fear of failure. Several questions aid this process, and readers can refer to the end of this chapter for a suggested team meeting agenda and to chapter 7 (section II, step 2) for an exercise designed for this purpose. After this has been completed, share the future state characteristics and stretch goals with the executive sponsor of the creative idea committee and suggest that time be devoted at a future committee meeting to discuss them. The sponsor also may feel it appropriate to share them with the CEO, the medical staff, and the governing board.

2. Define the Project

A shared vision of the future state, a world-class medication management process, is a critical first step in constructing projects to achieve the stretch goals.

However, organizations tend to rush too quickly into solutions without attempting to define the project's measurable impact on a subprocess. Therefore, a definition of a project is critical at this juncture. A project is a time-limited, process-outcome-oriented, measurable activity involving the implementation of one or more process changes. It is not the implementation of the change itself. For example, a project is not "to implement handheld medication ordering devices on 3w, Neuro, and Perinatal." That is a change.

A project would be to "reduce ordering errors by X percent in six months." Thus, the project involves one or more changes, such as installing handheld devices, in addition to limiting the choices of strengths and concentrations of selected drugs and deployment of guided-dose algorithm tools.

The reason for this critical distinction has been pointed out by Tom Nolan over the years. He has observed that "not all changes result in an improvement" (Nolan 2000). Therefore, tracking the result of a single change or multiple changes and implementations is an important feature of the 100-Day Plan process.

However, it is not inappropriate to designate a change or changes within a project charter. As above, for example, the medication error team might state that the project scope is "to reduce ordering errors by X percent in six months through the implementation of handheld devices on 3w, Neuro, and Perinatal."

3. Determine the Team

Another important concept related to projects is that not all projects need to be handled by a team. In the quality improvement (QI) structures of the 1990s, it was often taught that all projects require a team. Some projects, however, can be carried out more quickly by a single manager or perhaps a team of only two or three. Assigning projects to individuals and allowing them to determine the necessity for the involvement of others is a major accelerator to your work. However, it is also important that those affected by potential process changes be involved in some way so that the negative effect of surprise process changes on key stakeholders does not disrupt implementation.

As team members visualize the future state and stretch goals, allow them to brainstorm as many project ideas as possible. Most team members will have some experience with potential project ideas from past implementations and discussions at conferences and with colleagues. In addition, many articles and books are providing an exceptional database of ideas. Chapter 5 includes many ideas from the work of the IHI and others leading the medication error reduction effort.

4. Assess the Impact of Each Project

After a full list of potential projects has surfaced, the team can assess the potential effect of each project. Using the estimated project selection matrix in Figure 4.9, or a similar tool in active use in the organization, the team can estimate how to derive the most "bang for the buck." The medication error team leader should complete a draft for reaction by the team,

FIGURE 4.9.   PROJECT SELECTION MATRIX

Medication Error 3-Year Stretch Goals and Potential Projects

Medication Error 3-Year Stretch Goals and Potential Projects	50% Medication Error Reduction	50% ADE Reduction	Med Error Team Members Achieve "4" or "5" Each Month	Reduce Medication Cost per Discharge 20%
Medication error team members implement one change concept per month in 12 months.	High (impact) 30–90 (days until impact)	High 30–90	High 30–90	Low 30–90
In collaboration with the surgical errors team, reduce administration errors by 50% by deploying bedside medical error mitigation devices, such as Bridge Medical, in 9 months.	High 90–180	High 90–180		Moderate >180
Achieve 90% path use rate for included drugs in 12 months for the top 10 DRGS.	Moderate 90–180	Moderate 90–180	Low 90–180	Moderate 90–180
Reduce drug–patient misidentification errors by 75% and known allergy errors by 50% through implementation of bar coding to match drugs to patient wrist bands within 6 months.	High >180	High >180		Moderate >180
Reduce ordering errors by 50% through deployment of handheld ordering devices on 3W, neuro, and critical care in 4 months.	High 90–180	High 90–180	Low 90–180	High >180
Reduce dangerous drug errors by 50% by removing KCl from floor stock (again) and other interventions, and audit for compliance every quarter.	High 30–90	High 30–90		Moderate 30–90

Reprinted with permission. Chip Caldwell & Associates, LLC.

as opposed to completing the matrix in a team meeting. This type of pre-work is an effective technique for speeding up the deployment process and does not hamper team performance or cohesiveness unless the team leader is too forceful in driving consensus.

5. Determine How Many Projects to Charter

The number of projects undertaken simultaneously depends on the number of other initiatives under way in the organization and the significance of medication error reduction to executive management. As a general rule, however, each manager can actively manage one project at a time. If at all possible, managers should resist serving as team members on other projects. They should, however, provide ad hoc assistance, telephone consultation, or other forms of support as needed. Likewise, managers serving as project leaders should avoid requesting the active engagement of other managers except when they are truly needed. An organization with 20 managers making up the medication management system should be able to expect that 20 projects, each implementing one change per month, will be deployed at any given time.

6. Organize and Plan the Charter Projects

After team members have agreed on the projects to charter, the next step is to select project leaders and any support staff, agree on the project charters and measures, and set the start dates and anticipated completion dates.

Project leaders then plan their projects and provide input to the 100-Day Plan project planner, indicating major steps, start dates, and key milestone dates. All projects and their milestone dates are then included in the medication error team's 100-Day Plan project planner by the medication error team leader for monitoring by the creative idea committee.

The match staffing to demand team, being a shadow function of the medication error team and other patient safety teams, follows a somewhat more structured path to goal achievement. Because its charter is to convert 70 percent (or more) of time saved into productivity gains, this team is dependent on projects completed by the other teams.

Leveraging Step 2 for Success

To optimize the effectiveness of the tasks in step 2, consider the following:

- Do not delay while searching for the "perfect" data or source of data.
- Avoid collecting data on every conceivable control variable.

- Set true stretch goals, not simply what is conceivable at the moment.
- Be diligent in constructing project milestone dates and in using the 100-Day Plan project planner. This ensures that the medication error team and, ultimately, the creative idea team, stays on track and that the current position relative to the goal is known at critical times during the initiative.
- Convert the match staffing to demand team's ability to creatively recapture lost productivity regained by patient safety teams into true, bottom-line benefits for the organization's customers.

STEP 3. IMPLEMENT IDEALIZED DESIGN CHANGE CONCEPTS

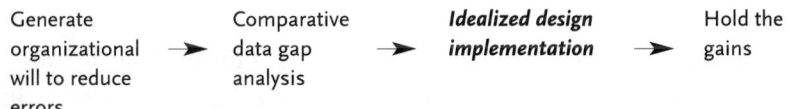

Both Mike Slubowski, an exceptional executive from Trinity Health System headquartered in Farmington Hills, Michigan, and Phil Beauchamp, CEO of Morton Plan Mease Health System in Dunedin, Florida, shared a *Fortune* magazine article with us in mid-1999 that polled CEOs from several large, successful American companies such as GE, Alcoa, IBM, and Cisco. The article probed for insights from these captains of large-scale change about how they had achieved unparalleled success in their respective companies. Some spoke of vision, some of commitment, and some of listening to the customer—the kinds of things one might expect. However, one factor was universal, a characteristic so basic that its simplicity rang of profoundness. That factor was a relentless focus on execution—yet, this factor, as each acknowledged, is so often overlooked.

In all the stories we collected in preparation for this book, no magic bullets were shared, no wonderful new organizational structures created, and no breakthrough tools innovated. Rather, the characteristics of simply staying the course, rewarding those who get things done, and committing to do what was promised appeared in every case study. Observations across multiple companies, inside and outside healthcare, point to the fact that when performance slips, the urge of senior management is to charter more teams, exert more effort, and demand that managers work harder. In fact, one large industrial client we worked with in the mid-1990s had created more than 90 action teams to get back to budget! The last of these teams were estimated to create only a few thousand dollars in incremental earnings for this multibillion dollar company. Yet, the highly leveraged teams were floundering without additional support and without a full analysis of the root causes of their slippage.

The intent of the 100-Day Plan management method (and, specifically, step 3) is to help executives and managers stay focused on implementation, reserving time to plan additional projects for specified periods within the 21-day planning windows.

Change Concepts

The field of quality improvement and cost reduction has enjoyed less success in implementing benchmarked processes and replicating best practices from other institutions than has been experienced in other industries. The reasons for this dilemma are varied, but one main factor is the belief among physicians and other professional groups that healthcare is somehow "different."

One response to this attitude is to cut through the underlying causes of our inability to replicate specific process changes discovered at other institutions. The methodology innovated by IHI in its Breakthrough Series approach, referenced so many times in this book, was found by the authors to be the most effective in terms of total effect on adverse drug events and medication errors and on the speed of implementation. One of the reasons for its success is the way in which potential change ideas are introduced into the organization. Rather than espouse a single solution, such as "remove KCI from floor stock," potential changes or ideas are assembled into common groupings called *change concepts* (Leape et al. 1998). For this example, the change concept would be "use constraints and forcing functions." Chapter 5 includes a listing of change concepts that have proven effective in reducing adverse drug events and medication errors.

The reason the application of change concepts works so much better than advocating a specific change is that the "not invented here" argument is immediately eliminated. Instead, an idealized design construct, such as forcing functions or standardization, is placed in front of the team and the team is given the flexibility and freedom to creatively adapt potential changes to its working environment. The team is given total control, rather than having control taken away from it. The only caveat for the team is that status quo is not an option. Many specific recommended changes will elicit a barrage of reasons why they will not be effective in the organization. Using the change concept approach, this is an acceptable reaction as long as the status quo is not maintained. The team can modify an existing change or choose to innovate a new one, as long as some change is executed quickly.

Therefore, the definition of a *change* is "a specific idea, best practice, or other process modification that can be implemented to achieve a reduction in adverse drug events and medication errors," for example, "color code the wristbands of patients with allergies" (Leape et al. 1998). A *change concept* is a category or grouping of changes, for example, "Improve access to information," which is the change concept for the color-coding suggestion above.

Each project uses the idealized design implementation process to identify or construct a database of ideas, implement them, and monitor progress. The idealized design implementation step involves three tasks:

1. Search or create change concepts databases in the knowledge management loop.
2. Implement 30-day cycle aim-measure-PDSA ramps.
3. Track to ensure that projects stay on schedule.

Search or Create Change Concepts Databases in the Knowledge Management Loop

Many change concepts exist for medication error reduction from which each project can draw. This is not the case for other medical error categories such as surgical errors and critical care errors. For specific change concepts for medication error reduction, refer to chapter 5 of this book, the IHI materials, and the ISMP and other research organizations that are devoting significant effort to producing innovate process changes that can be input into the 100-Day Plan methodology.

In the absence of a credible change concepts database, or to introduce new change concepts, the project leader must execute the knowledge management loop by creating a new database. For example, to attack drug use through enhanced clinical paths, the project leader would establish a change concepts database, as suggested in the estimated project selection matrix in Figure 4.9.

The first step in creating the database is to retain the services of an outside subject matter expert (SME) to lead the internal effort, supported by the project leader and the facilitator. The SME need not come from outside the IDN; however, an inside resource, although credible, is less likely to be as successful.

Second, in an effort to construct an evidence-based change concepts database, the SME will assemble available literature and, if possible, the names of one or more benchmark organizations. A site visit to at least one of these organizations can be very effective. After this is completed, the project leader and the facilitator can construct the ideas into a change concepts database by organizing them into groupings. For a complete listing of change concepts, refer to the appendix in *The Improvement Guide* (Langley et al. 1996).

Implement 30-Day Cycle Aim-Measure-PDSA Ramps

After a credible change concepts database has been acquired or created by the project leader, the process of implementation begins. Each project leader is expected to implement one change per month, or in the case of a very large project requiring more than six months (for example, implementation of a bedside medication error mitigation technology), to complete a major milestone each month. However, large projects should not become a crutch to slow implementation.

To record the time saved by each change implemented, an important process for each project leader chartered by the medication error team is to complete the process analysis spreadsheet, illustrated in Table 4.1. This information is vital to the work of the match staffing to demand team. In the absence of these data, the match staffing to demand team must rework much of the medication error team's project to recapture the amount of lost productivity gained from its process change.

The match staffing to demand team acquires completed process analysis spreadsheets from each project leader and engages match staffing to demand change concepts, discussed in chapter 6, to convert this lost productivity into measurable results.

Track to Ensure That Projects Stay on Schedule

At the end of each month, each project leader self-scores his or her activity for the month according to the 5-to-1 scale discussed in Figure 4.8, as follows:

1 = No activity
2 = Activity, no strategic results
3 = Activity, time saved, but no cost recaptured
4 = Activity, time saved, one-time cost recaptured (e.g., inventory reduction)
5 = Activity, time saved, sustainable cost recaptured (e.g., FTE reduction)

An example of the project leader activity results report card is shown in Figure 4.10.

This self-scoring is validated by the medication errors team leader and all project leader scores for the month are aggregated to form the monthly medication error team activity results report card. (See Figure 4.8.)

Recapture Lost Productivity and Cost

Central to the 100-Day Plan method is the conversion of the time saved as a result of error reduction. If the average organization is wasting up to 10

TABLE 4.1.   PROCESS ANALYSIS WORKSHEET

Process Name (and boundaries):

Process Owner(s):

Step No. (1)	Activity (2)	Responsible Position (3)	Volume per Week (4)	No. of Individuals (5)	Total Hours per Week (6)	NVA (Y/N?) (7)	NVA Hours per Week (8)
Sum=							

Chip Caldwell (ed). 1998. *The Handbook for Managing Change in Healthcare.* Milwaukee, WI: ASQ Quality Press, 272. Copyright Chip Caldwell & Associates, LLC. 2001.

FIGURE 4.10.   PROJECT LEADER ACTIVITY RESULTS REPORT CARD,
ALLERGY ERROR REDUCTION PROJECT

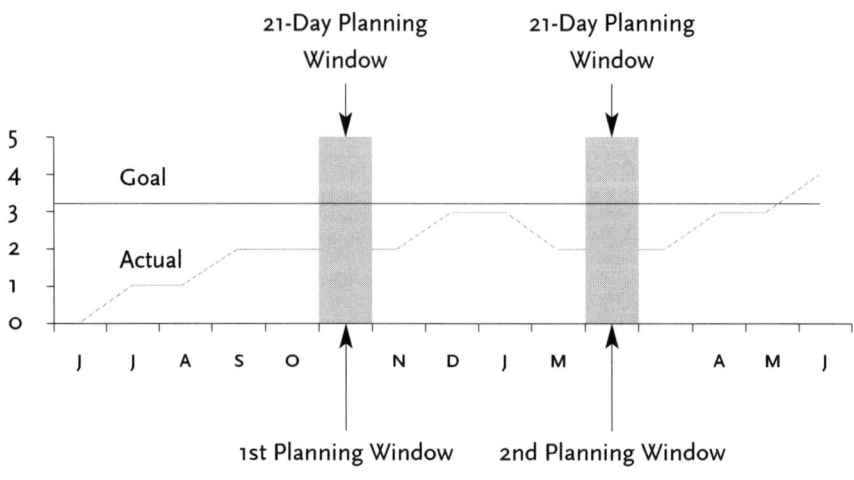

Reprinted with permission. Chip Caldwell & Associates, LLC.

percent of total medication management iterations, as held by Leape, Bates
and others, a significant amount of time is being wasted. As adverse drug
events and medication errors are decreased, the effect is to free up time consumed by lost productivity (see Figure 4.11).

This recapture, however, is not automatic. The organization must take
specific actions to realize the recapture of productivity lost to poor quality.
In the 100-Day Plan management method, this duty falls to the match
staffing to demand team (Figure 4.5). This recapture also requires the implementation of defined tactics, referred to as the match staffing to demand
change concepts (discussed in detail in chapter 6).

Leveraging Step 3 for Success

Listed below are several leverage points revealed by the IHI (Leape et al.
1998) and Caldwell (1995):

- Resist straying from the original aim.
- Set aggressive stretch goals.
- Avoid too many or ineffective measures.

FIGURE 4.11.   RECAPTURING LOST PRODUCTIVITY

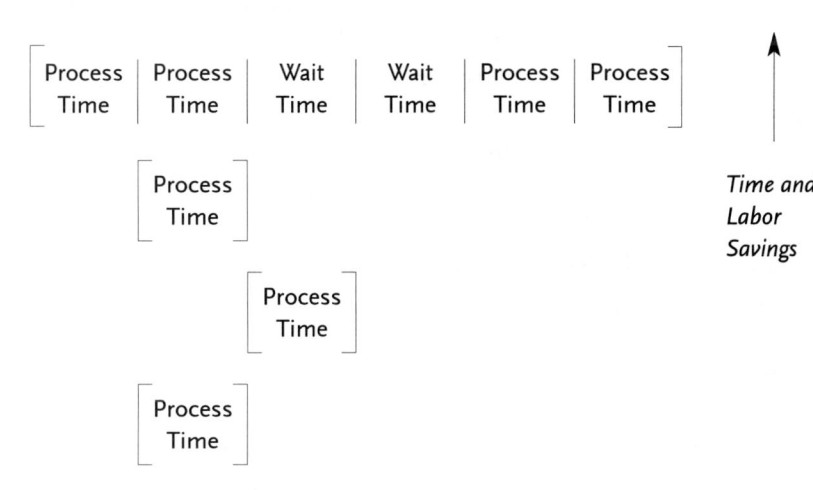

- Do not wait for information systems to provide the measure; use sampling when manual collection is required.
- To ensure momentum, craft plans for the next two to three cycles (Caldwell 1995).
- Select changes that are acceptable to the majority.
- Strive to learn and improve the process after each cycle (Caldwell 1995).
- If it can't be tested within the next 30 days, move on to the next idea.
- Steal shamelessly from others.
- Engage in defined activity to recapture lost productivity and cost to convert error reduction into bottom-line savings.

STEP 4. HOLD THE GAINS

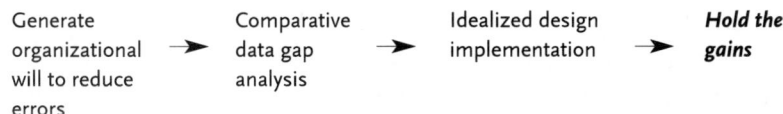

The last step in the 100-Day Plan management system is to hold the gains. This step is what Juran called "hand-off to operations." In his quality management trilogy—quality planning, quality improvement, and quality control—it was his position that as QI cycles were completed, the QI team either disbanded or was chartered into another improvement cycle. Maintaining the improvements was then incorporated into the day-to-day procedures of operating departments and executive management. He urged managers to ensure that changes "held the gain" as quality control, believing it is the managers' responsibility, not the team's, to periodically monitor the changes.

Likewise, we agree that individual managers and executives should take over the function of periodically monitoring process changes to ensure that the new level of performance is maintained.

To accomplish step 4, it is necessary to monitor the balanced scorecard and stabilize the gain.

Monitor the Balanced Scorecard

After progress in the reduction of adverse drug events and medication errors has been made over time by the medication error team and the creative idea committee, thresholds in the balanced scorecard should be adjusted to ensure that any slippage in performance becomes immediately apparent.

Stabilize the Gain

A management engineer or other capable individual within the organization should be deployed to help operating managers periodically audit process changes to ensure that gains are held. If critical, such as allergy mishaps, these measures can be incorporated into the manager's monthly strategic measurement set.

Leveraging Step 4 for Success

Consider the following factors when looking to optimize the tasks in step 4:

- Adjust balanced scorecard thresholds to accommodate the new level of performance.
- Audit, at the department level, to ensure that gains are held.
- Review manager audit techniques at a monthly manager meeting so that learning of best practices occurs.

In conclusion, this 4-step, 100-Day Plan management method provides a disciplined, concise approach to the reduction of medication errors and the recovery of costs associated with them.

REFERENCES

Ackoff, R. 1999. *Re-Creating the Corporation*. New York: Oxford Press.

Agency for Healthcare Research and Quality. 2000. "20 Tips to Prevent Medical Errors." Available online at www.ahrq.gov/consumer/20tips.htm.

Bates, D.W., N. Spell, D.J. Cullen, E. Burdick, N. Laird, L.A. Petersen, S.D. Small, B.J. Sweitzer, and L.L. Leape. 1997. "The Costs of Adverse Drug Events in Hospitalized Patients." *Journal of the American Medical Association* 277: 307–11.

Caldwell, C. 1995. *Mentoring Strategic Change in Health Care*. Milwaukee, WI: ASQ Quality Press.

Clinical Initiatives Center. 1999. *Prescription for Change: Toward a Higher Standard in Medication Management*. Washington, D.C.: The Advisory Board Company.

Cohen, M. 1998. "Survey of Hospital Systems and Common Serious Medication Errors." *Journal of Healthcare Risk Management* 18(1): 16–28.

James, B. 1999. *Personal interview*. Salt Lake City, November 4.

Kelly, L. 1999. *How to Use Control Charts for Healthcare*. Milwaukee, WI: ASQ Quality Press. Available online at www.asq.org.

Kizer, K. 2000. "Scope of Medical Error Problem." Paper presented at Premier CEO-M.D. Leadership Forum, Tyson Corners, VA, April 18.

Langley, G., K. Nolan, T. Nolan, C. Norman, and L. Provost. 1996. *The Improvement Guide*. San Francisco: Jossey-Bass.

Leape, L., A. Kabcenell, D. Berwick, and J. Roessner. 1998. *Reducing Adverse Drug Events*. Boston: Institute for Healthcare Improvement.

Leape, L., T. Brennan, N. Laird, A.G. Lawthers, A. R. LoCalio, B.A. Barnes, L. Hebert, J.P. Newhouse, P.C. Weiler, and H. Hiatt. 1991. "The Nature of Adverse Events in Hospitalized Patients: Results of the Harvard Medical Practice Study II." *New England Journal of Medicine* 324(6): 377–84.

National Health Information. 2000. "Self-benchmarking Improves Care, Cuts Drug Errors." *Data Strategies and Benchmarks*. Atlanta: National Health Information.

Nolan, T. 2000. "Institute for Healthcare Improvement Breakthrough Series Results." Paper presented at Premier Rapid Response Forum, Charlotte, NC, February 17.

Premier, Inc. 1994. *Foundation Statement*. San Diego, CA: Premier, Inc.

Reinertsen, J. 2000. "Addressing Medication Errors." Paper presented at Premier CEO-M.D. Leadership Forum, Tyson Corners, VA, April 18.

Ryan, M.J. 2000. Interview with the author, March 3.

Spreadbury, B. 2000. Interview with the author, Charlotte, NC, April 10.

Stepanovich, P., and J. Uhrig. 1999. "Decision Making in High-Velocity Environments: Implications for Healthcare." *Journal of Healthcare Management* 44(3): 197–205.

Welch, J. 1996. "Success at GE." Paper Presented at Premier CEO Invitational Meeting, Aspen, CO, July 15.

Womack, J., D. Jones, and D. Roos. 1990. *The Machine That Changed the World.* New York: Harper Perennial.

Yasuda, Y. 1991. *40 Years, 20 Million Ideas: The Toyota Suggestion System.* Cambridge, MA: Productivity Press.

QUESTIONS FOR A ONE-HOUR EXECUTIVE MEETING

During this first review session, executives should assess the effectivness of the organization's measurement process.

1. Review the organization's balanced scorecard for the presence of effective safety-related measures.
2. Look for measures linked to risk management issues and areas of highest incidence of medical errors (medication errors, surgical errors, nosocomial infections, anesthesia accidents, etc.).
3. If more than 15 measures exist, discuss the removal of subordinate measures from the balanced scorecard and place them on the appropriate vice president's measurement set. For example, if the balanced scorecard contains supply costs per discharge (or supply costs as a percent of total operating costs) and total cost per discharge (or operating cost as a percent of net revenue), consider moving supply chain or other cost measures to the CFO's measurement set.
4. For measures available only semiannually or annually, such as patient satisfaction, discuss proxy measures that may be available more frequently, such as complaints per 100 discharges.

QUESTIONS FOR A ONE-HOUR MEDICATION ERROR TEAM MEETING

During the first and second sessions, the team should envision the future state of the medication management process. Some team members will embrace this world-class state with vigor; others will allow the fear of failure to overcome them. It is vital to ultimate success that all team members share a vision of the future state and understand what changes will be required. Devoted team time may aid this process.

1. Meeting prework:
   a. In advance of the meeting, record the vision on a flip chart and tape it to the wall.
   b. Record the three-year stretch goals and tape them to the wall.
   c. Draw the high-level flowchart from the exercise above and tape it to the wall.
2. On a blank flip chart, ask team members to brainstorm characteristics of the current state of the medication management system. You may prefer to use a cause-and-effect diagram to stimulate characteristics for all key components of the system. In the absence

of a cause-and-effect diagram, ensure that characteristics are present for:

- people in the system (caregivers, management and executive staff, physicians, support staff);
- processes (procedures, policies, guidelines, clinical paths, formulary);
- systems (IT, robotics, medical records, admitting, staff scheduling);
- environment (managed care and Medicare requirements, regulatory requirements);
- beliefs about adverse drug events and medication errors and the medication management process; and
- any other critical categories.

3. Next, ask team members to brainstorm characteristics of a medication management system achieving the three-year goals, again making sure to cover key categories: "In a medication management system that produces only X% errors, what would be the characteristics of the system, of our staff and physicians, and of our IT environment?"

4. After the meeting, clarify and summarize these future state characteristics.

5. At a future meeting, discuss again the implications, barriers, attractiveness, and supports of the future state. Attempt to come up with a one- to two-sentence descriptor of the future state and put it in front of the team often.

QUESTIONS FOR A ONE-HOUR GOVERNING BODY MEETING

1. Review the medication error team's 100-Day Plan, project selection matrix, and monthly activity results report card, and the specifics of one project.

2. Allow members to comment, based on their experience in other industries or knowledge gained from discussions with colleagues at other institutions.

CHAPTER FIVE

Knowledge Management Loop for Medication Error Reduction

I cannot say whether things will get better if we change;
what I can say is they must change if they are to get better.

—G. C. Lichtenberg

T HIS CHAPTER PROVIDES several change concepts from recognized sources in the area of medical error and medication error reduction.

A PROCESS FOR SELECTING AND PRIORITIZING CHANGE CONCEPTS

The knowledge management loop, nested inside step 3 of the 100-Day Plan management method, produces an evidence-based database of change concepts for implementation throughout the IDN or medical center. These databases are not static but, rather, require periodic revitalization as creative idea teams charter projects to implement them. As discussed in chapter 4, the database is created under the guidance of a knowledgeable expert called the subject matter expert (SME). The SME is retained by the organization to spend several days on-site to work with the project leader and the facilitator and, in circumstances where there is significant resistance to change, perhaps directly with the key stakeholders (physicians, nurses, and other staff). The SME researches available literature and conducts process-benchmarking interviews to uncover additional ideas for implementation by project teams. As ideas are implemented or creatively modified to produce an alternate process change, the project leader will see the need to revitalize and upgrade the change concepts database.

However, most organizations will not need to kick off their initiatives with the engagement of an SME because they already will have identified a sufficient number of change concepts to initiate the 100-Day Plan implementation process. This is particularly true in the case of medication error change concepts. A rich set of change concepts, constantly growing and widely shared, appears robust enough to sustain most IDNs and medical centers for up to 12 months.

Before revealing several change concepts from reputable experts in the area of medication error reduction, the 100-Day Plan management method requires consideration of some additional concepts that will aid in prioritizing and measuring the ultimate long-term effect of implemented process changes.

First, as discussed in chapter 4, we advocate attacking adverse drug events and medication errors not by drug type or adverse drug event consequence but, rather, by process failures handled through logical work teams. Changes should be implemented by individuals who make up a work group within a preexisting, defined area, such as a department or clinical path. Typically, such individuals—physicians, nurses, respiratory therapists, pharmacists, and so on—have worked together on a day-to-day basis and will continue to do so after a project has achieved its goals. Their culture of working together enables them to accelerate the implementation of projects in a way that a newly formed project team would be unable to do. Further, as the work group completes one set of goals, its members are uniquely positioned to take on another project. They learn to work better together over time and to manage the consequences of successful and unsuccessful changes on a day-to-day basis.

Second, we encourage the prioritizing of projects, using the project selection matrix discussed in chapter 4, based on each project's potential effect on strategies, high error-prone processes, and speed of deployment. Rather than beginning by implementing changes within all subprocesses of the medication management system (prescribing, ordering, dispensing, administration, and monitoring), we advocate sharpening the saw prior to goal and project selection based on the potential effect on key strategies.

There are several possible dimensions to assess in prioritizing the subprocesses for attention, most notably by:

- adverse event frequency;
- total medication error frequency;
- cost effect (malpractice indemnity payments, malpractice cost, recovery cost, cost of quality assurance, and lost productivity cost);
- drug class;
- high-risk drug and/or patient class; and
- subprocess effect.

A set of data elements extractable from the literature for analysis and easily supplemented by IDN or facility data, if desired, includes:

- compensable event cost (malpractice indemnity payments, both court awarded and out-of-court settlements).
- potential compensable event cost (malpractice claims cost, including attorney fees, investigation cost, staff time to analyze adverse events that could be deployed to patient care activities using the match staffing to demand change concepts discussed in chapter 6, and an estimate of indirect costs).
- defensive medicine cost, which, according to one study, approaches 8 percent of total diagnostic procedures (U.S. House 1995).
- adverse drug event costs (including investigation costs; cost of error detection; staff time to analyze adverse events that could be deployed to patient care activities; remedy costs to patients and families; remedy process costs to detect future occurrences such as added inspection and staff education; and time and productivity cost for medical staff and management committees and all the staff hours that support them that could be redirected or eliminated).
- medication error costs (including all subprocess costs that must be reworked, such as additional prescribing time and physician lost productivity cost; additional order time and nursing productivity cost; additional dispensing supply cost, time, and pharmacist productivity cost; nurse administration time and productivity cost; and nurse monitoring time and productivity cost).
- near-miss costs, including the costs above.

Many of the categories of cost listed above are the result of lost productivity. It is worth repeating at this point that the rescue of the American automobile industry in the 1980s and 1990s rested on dramatically improving quality while recapturing lost productivity. The notion of six sigma depends on the premise that at three sigma, or 66,807 errors per one million opportunities, the cost of quality is about 25 to 40 percent of total costs, whereas the cost of quality for six sigma, or 3.4 errors per one million opportunities, is immeasurable (Harry and Schroder 1999). Extrapolating from Leape's occurrence data places medication errors close to 2.5 sigma (Leape et al. 1995). Calculating the cost of quality at this level suggests that the typical healthcare organization expends between 25 and 40 percent of its total operating budget on adverse drug events and medication errors—those costs delineated above. Recovery of these costs requires additional process changes and is discussed in greater detail in Chapter 6 "Knowledge Management Loop to Match Staffing to Demand."

Some of these costs have been reported in the literature and can serve to guide initial prioritization. From a malpractice insurance cost perspective, the stakes remain quite high. St. Paul Fire and Marine conducted an analysis in 1994 of the average malpractice rates per bed by major metropolitan area, as follows (U.S. House 1995):

Metropolitan Area	Per Bed Rate
Detroit	$7,734
Kansas City	$4,472
St. Louis	$4,472
Los Angeles	$4,114
New York	$3,424
Miami	$3,367
Chicago	$3,309
San Francisco	$2,797
Cleveland	$2,467
Richmond	$1,113

Although easing insurance costs requires more than a year for actuarial data to affect the trended cost formula, these costs cannot go unnoticed.

The classes of drugs driving the highest percentage of claims also are fairly certain. In an analysis of claims through 1979, the Insurance Company of North America found that almost 6 percent of total claims were drug related, which did not take into account incorrect patient information. The company reported that the basis of drug-related claims were (Fink 1983):

Basis	Percent
Side effects	54.3
Incorrect drug	26.5
Misdosing	14.5

Further, in a more recent study concluded in 1997, 60 percent of claims were associated with five drug classes, as follows (Dwyer 1998):

- antibiotics;
- anticoagulants;
- steroids;
- narcotics; and
- cardiovascular.

FIGURE 5.1. PROCESS-FOCUSED PRIORITIZATION FLOWCHART

	Physician ➤ Prescribing	Order ➤ Processing	Drug ➤ Preparation	Drug ➤ Administration	Drug Monitoring
Occurrence Percent	39 %	12 %	11 %	38 %	NA
Percent Interrupted	48 %	33 %	34 %	2 %	NA
Potential Productivity Recapture	High	Medium	Low	High	High

In work reported by the Cleveland Clinic in 2000, the following occurrence error percentages were found by drug class (Clough 2000):

Antibiotics	19
CNS drugs	18
Cardiovascular	13
Fluid and electrolytes	8
Anticoagulants	7
Diuretics	5
Insulin	4
Other	24

Using this information and similar data reported in this book, a process-focused viewpoint can help stimulate prioritization (see Figure 5.1).

Based on a process orientation to medication error reduction, it would seem most logical to initially focus efforts on those errors occurring in the ordering subprocess because this is where most adverse drug events occur. Further, the ability to recapture lost productivity in this process and the downstream monitoring subprocess is highest. The activities and tasks within the ordering process with the highest leverage points are (Leape et al. 1995):

- lack of drug knowledge (29 percent);
- dose and patient identify checking (12 percent); and
- patient information availability, including allergy (11 percent).

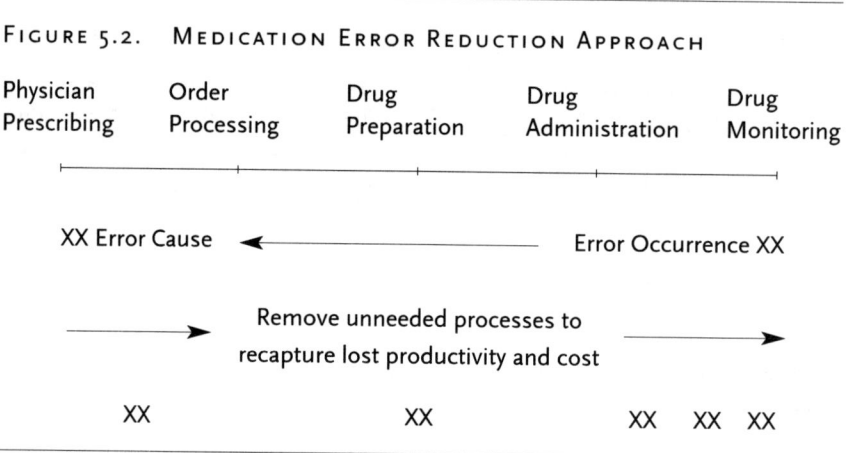

FIGURE 5.2.   MEDICATION ERROR REDUCTION APPROACH

| Physician Prescribing | Order Processing | Drug Preparation | Drug Administration | Drug Monitoring |

XX Error Cause ◄─────────────── Error Occurrence XX

─────────► Remove unneeded processes to
recapture lost productivity and cost ─────────►

XX   XX   XX   XX   XX

The intervention approach to both reduce errors and regain lost productivity resulting from errors (discussed again in chapter 6) is illustrated in Figure 5.2.

After the locus of the error is determined, it is possible to move upstream and locate the precise subprocess and activity or task-level cause of the error. Using the medication error reduction change concepts database, the project leader can introduce changes that eliminate or dramatically reduce the potential for recurrence. Then, using the process analysis spreadsheet shown in Table 4.1, the project leader can determine which downstream steps to eliminate. The spreadsheet is then handed over to the match staffing to demand team, which can now work to convert those changes, and others to support them, into recaptured lost productivity for ultimate improvement in both quality and costs.

Following this prioritization logic enables the IDN and/or medical center to optimize deployment of change concepts and the resources and energy devoted to medication error reduction.

CHANGE CONCEPTS FOR MEDICATION ERROR REDUCTION

More change concepts exist for the reduction of medication error than perhaps any other type of medical error. Although these changes have been proposed for a number of years, few showcase sites can be found where widespread concentration on medication error reduction has been a strategic focus. None have been found that have successfully recaptured the associated lost productivity from adverse drug events and medication errors. The next two sections list change concepts developed by the Institute for Safe Medication Practices (ISMP) and the Institute for Healthcare Improvement (IHI), two organizations with vast experience in medication error reduction.

Institute for Safe Medication Practices

The Institute for Safe Medication Practices, located in Huntington, Pennsylvania, in collaboration with the American Hospital Association (AHA), produced a self-assessment tool that suggests specific process changes (ISMP 2000). The self-assessment approach is an effective way to prioritize potential process changes. Several elements of the ISMP approach follow.

- Is essential patient information available when prescribing, dispensing, and administering medications?
  -Allergy information is required prior to ordering.
  -Automated computer screening is done to determine allergic potential.
  -Bar coding is used.
  -Monitoring criteria have been standardized.
  -Pharmacy system and lab system interfaces have been made to automatically alert staff to medication changes.
- Is drug information available when prescribing, ordering, dispensing, and administering medications?
  -Patient's complete medication history is needed.
  -Maximum doses for high-risk drugs are specified.
  -Computer system automatically checks dose ranges.
- Has a closed drug formulary system been established to limit choice to essential drugs, minimize the number of drugs with which practitioners must be familiar, and provide adequate time to design safe processes for the use of new drugs added to the formulary?
  -No duplicate generic equivalents exist.
  -The potential for adverse events is considered prior to adding a drug to the formulary.
- Are methods of communicating drug orders and other drug information standardized and automated to minimize the risk of error?
  -Prescribers enter orders directly into the pharmacy system.
  -Standardized formats for abbreviations and doses exist.
  -Orders to follow the current therapy regime upon patient unit transfers are not accepted.
- Have processes been implemented to reduce sound-alike, look-alike errors?
  -Look-alike drugs are kept separately rather than alphabetically.

-Redundant warnings are in use.

-The clinical indication is included on orders to aid error prevention and detection.

- Are clear and readable labels that identify drugs on all drug containers, and do drugs remain labeled up to the point of actual drug administration?
- Are IV solutions, drug concentrations, doses, and administration times standardized?
- Are medications delivered to patient care units in a safe and secure manner and available for administration within a time frame that meets essential patient needs?
- Is unit-based floor stock appropriately restricted?
- Are hazardous chemicals safely stored away from patients and inaccessible in drug preparation areas?
- Is the potential for human error mitigated through careful procurement, maintenance, use, and standardization of medication delivery devices?
- Are medications prescribed, transcribed, prepared, dispensed, and administered in a physical environment that offers adequate space and lighting and allows practitioners to remain focused on medication use without distractions?
- Does the complement of qualified, well-rested practitioners match the clinical workload without compromising patient safety?
- Do practitioners receive sufficient orientation to medication use, and do they undergo baseline and annual competency evaluation of knowledge and skills related to safe medication practices?
- Are practitioners involved in medication use provided with ongoing education about medication error prevention and the safe use of drugs that have the greatest potential to cause harm if misused?
- Are patients included as active partners in their care through education about their medications and ways to avert errors?
- Is a nonpunitive, system-based approach to error reduction in place?
- Are practitioners stimulated to detect and report errors, and do multidisciplinary teams regularly analyze errors that have occurred within the organization and in other organizations for the purpose of redesigning systems to better support safe practitioner performance?
- Are redundancies in place to support a system of independent double-checks, or is an automated verification process used for vulnerable parts of the medication system to detect and correct serious errors before they reach patients?
- Are proven infection control practices followed when storing, preparing, and administering medications?

Institute for Healthcare Improvement

This section lists proven remedies from *Reducing Adverse Drug Events* (Leape et al. 1998), published by the Institute for Healthcare Improvement (reprinted here with permission of the publisher).

Standardize

- Standardize prescribing conventions
  -use no abbreviations
  -use "units" vs. "u"; use leading zero [0.5 not 5], but avoid trailing zero [5 not 5.0]
  -use generic names
  -use metric system only
  -do not use Q or q
  -use protocols and standing orders for complex medication administration (heparin, insulin, chemotherapy)
- Limit the number of standard doses of medication
- Standardize times of drug administration
- Store medications in the same place in every medication room
- Standardize packaging and labeling for all medications
- Make "like" drugs look alike and different drugs that look different
- Use standard equipment
- Attempt to standardize on one kind of pump to decrease the potential for error resulting from skills required to manage multiple devices serving the same purpose and possibility of inventory miscues

Use automation

- Computerized order entry
- Handheld computer ordering devices to reduce reliance on physician memory and avoid transcription steps
- Computerized prescriber order entry that automatically transmits the physician's order to both the pharmacy and the nursing station
- Bar coding (to match drug bar code to patient wrist band bar code and to identify drugs)
- Computerized patient information (including allergy information)
- Computerized drug dispensing, use of timers or alarms
- Automated dispensing on the unit
- Computerized patient medical information systems that interface computerized laboratory systems with medication management systems

- Automatic drug dose checking in high-risk situations
- Electronic monitors that signal an alarm when parameters are exceeded
- Computerized order entry systems with range checks and override capacity
- Robotic dispensing systems in the pharmacy
- Computerized medication administration record generated by the pharmacy

Reduce reliance on memory and attention

- Use drug-drug interaction checking systems
- Use guided dose algorithms
- Laminate dosing cards to help remember tasks
- Rotate staff when performing repetitive functions
- Deploy pocket formularies

Simplify processes

- Eliminate order transcription
- Limit choice of available drugs in pharmacy
- Limit the choices of dosage strengths and concentration for each drug
- Maintain inventory of frequently used prepared drugs, rather than preparing such drugs to order
- Limit the number of times per day that drugs are administrated, mix ivs in the pharmacy
- Use a single record entry for medications

Use constraints and forcing functions

- Design or select pharmacy computer systems that will not fill any orders unless allergy information and patient weight and height are entered
- Add special luer-locks to syringes and indwelling lines that have to match before fluid can be infused to prevent personnel from infusing non-iv solutions into ivs, central lines, or intrathecal lines
- Design or select computerized order systems with range checks on doses to prevent completion of an order until the dose specified is in a safe range for the medication and patient
- Remove concentrated potassium chloride solutions from floor stock, thus preventing accidental rapid iv infusion of a concentrated solution

Formalize the process

- Avoid statements that contain negatives in protocols and checklists (i.e., "check to see that the light is off" as opposed to "check to see that the light is not on")
- Make instructions agree with the most likely state of the system (so that a "yes" is the usual response)
- Verify regularly that everyone has agreed on the protocol or checklist to determine if exceptions exist that may require revision

Improve access to information

- Establish an ADE specialist staff person
- Create and share intervention database, managed by pharmacist or ADE specialist
- Assign the pharmacy or ADE specialist to create a computer database for intervention occurrences that can be shared for pharmacist, nurse, resident, and physician education; Pharmacy and Therapeutics Committee review; and other education and learning vehicles within the organization
- Have a pharmacist available on the nursing units and at rounds
- Design or select computerized order entry systems that provide easy access to drug and patient information
- Design or select computerized laboratory systems that immediately alert clinicians of abnormal lab values
- Place lab reports and medication records at the bedside
- Place protocols and ordering information on the patient's chart and in the medication room where they are easily accessible
- Color-code wristbands for patients with allergies
- Provide each patient with allergies with a list of his or her medications, doses, and times
- Track errors or near misses and report these to staff on a weekly basis
- Accelerate lab turnaround times for blood coagulation tests (partial thromboplastic time, or PTTs) and blood sugar tests

Optimize level of inspection

- Use double checks for doses of narcotics, insulin, heparin, chemotherapy, and other lethal drugs
- Establish high-risk rounding process
- Have the pharmacist monitor highly toxic drugs on a daily basis

- Conduct periodic quality audits to assure gains are held and protocols are in high use

Author's note: As the organization improves adverse drug events and medication errors through multiple improvement cycles, the potential for slipping back into previous habits or for introducing undesirable "work-around" habits increases. Evidence suggests that newly deployed checklists and any standardization with regard to times of administration will not maintain the initial level of conformance to requirements. One effective approach is an annual or semiannual audit to test for undesired variation. Such audits need not be as complex as the inspections done by the Joint Commission or others. Rather, they could be slightly sampled inspections in each department and functional area. Often it is not the actual variance that is important but, instead, the pre- and post-audit awareness generated as a result of the activity.

Reduce handoffs

- Provide ready-to-administer products
- Reduce transcription of medical orders
- Use unit-dosing systems and have a pharmacist participate in rounds
- Use automated point-of-care drug delivery systems
- Use computerized prescriber for order entry
- Use a satellite pharmacy

Author's note: The entire prescribing and ordering process, as it exists in most organizations, is fraught with the potential for error—from difficulty in reading the physician's handwriting to the number of steps involved in getting the prescription transmitted to the pharmacy. As discussed numerous times in this text, the greater the number of steps, the greater the likelihood that a mistake will occur.

Differentiate products

- Eliminate look-alikes and sound-alikes
- Repackage or relabel look-alike medications to differentiate them
- Store similar-looking medications in separate places
- Alert staff and post information on sound-alike medications
- Avoid sound-alikes by using the brand name for one medication and the generic name for the other
- Avoid stocking look-alike packages

Optimize the work environment for safety

- Keep workloads within an acceptable range
- Reduce unnecessary time pressure in any phase of the medication system
- Avoid double shifts and accommodate diurnal sleep rhythms
- Adjust the physician environment to increase light, decrease noise, and decrease clutter
- Keep critical equipment available; in good repair, and stored in a uniform manner
- Reduce distractions

Increase immediate feedback

- Use equipment that not only indicates there is a problem but also shows where the problem is
- Monitor the effectiveness of protocols instituted and provide information to all staff demonstrating the effectiveness of protocols
- Make staff aware of responses to reported errors

Train for teamwork

- Train leaders in a nonauthoritarian style of management and train workers to function as a team
- Train workers to be interdependent as well as independent
- Train for safety, emphasizing potential hazards and methods to avoid them
- Create stable teams to work with high-hazard substances
- Conduct regular small group discussions of "errors waiting to happen"
- Collect and disseminate information on common errors in the organization (i.e., feedback information to clinicians)
- Display run charts to show the effects of error reduction efforts (i.e., compliance with protocols, reduction of nonstandard orders, or automatic dose reduction for the elderly)

Emphasize natural and logical consequences

- Establish incentive plans for improvement

Move steps closer together

- Move MAR to the bedside

Remove demotivating aspects of error detection

- Publicly reward reports of error
- Establish safe havens for error reporting (i.e., grant immunity from punishment)
- Establish confidential reporting of errors
- Make error reporting easy (i.e., use simple forms)
- Display run charts to show increased reporting of errors

Consider people as in the same system

- Decrease competition and increase cooperation among staff
- Create interdisciplinary teams

Improve direct communication

- Train all staff to avoid indirect and mitigated communication
- Repeat verbal orders verbatim
- Role-play direct communication and methods for dealing with authoritarian style
- Provide feedback (including feedback in videotape format) about indirect and mitigated communication

Coach patients and families in the safe use of medications

- Provide patients and families with brochures and written instruction on the safe use of medication. Instruct them on how to help nurses check to assure the correct medication is being administered.
- Provide instruction on safe medication administration practices. HCAB reported that only 36 percent of physicians consistently instruct patients regarding the medication use (Clinical Initiatives Center 1999; Leape et al. 1998).

Deployment of the IHI Change Concepts

In 2000, Premier conducted a study of 38 healthcare organizations to assess their degree of deployment of the IHI change concepts. The data from this study are provided in Figure 5.3. (Those organizations interested in comparing themselves to this small study can complete the survey in section III of chapter 7.)

FIGURE 5.3.   MEDICATION ERROR CHANGE CONCEPT DEPLOYMENT

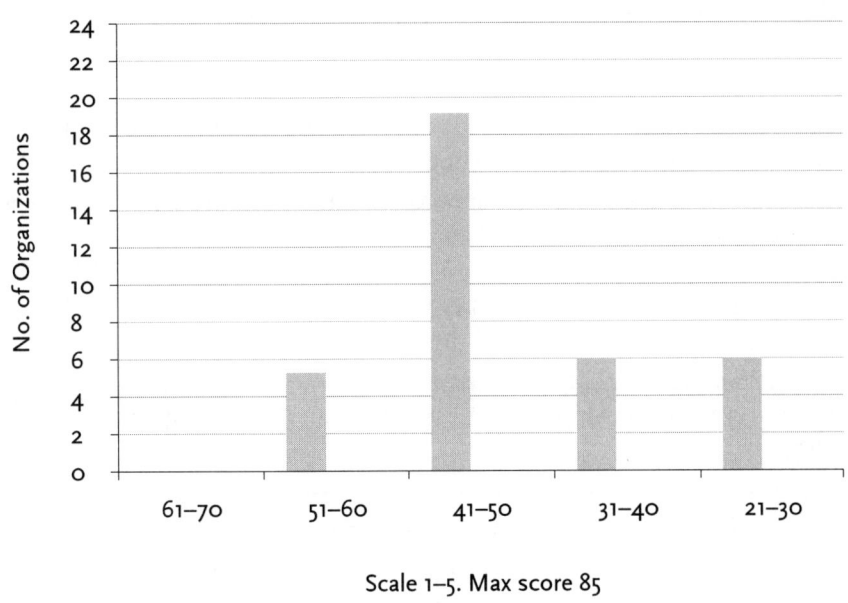

Scale 1–5. Max score 85

The greatest opportunities were found in the following areas, ranked in order:

1. automation;
2. multiple entries;
3. differentiation;
4. feedback systems;
5. communication;
6. protocols; and
7. information access.

Leape's Recommendations

Lucian Leape has suggested the following prioritization (Moore 1998):

1. Improve systems in which people work
2. Avoid reliance on memory

3. Simplify processes
4. Standardize
5. Use forcing functions
6. Use protocols and checklists wisely
7. Automate and use bar coding

In conclusion, these and other change concepts, in addition to implementation case studies, are actively published in the literature and serve as rich resources for the periodic updating of the organization's change concepts database.

REFERENCES

Clinical Initiatives Center. 1999. *Prescription for Change: Toward a Higher Standard in Medication Management.* Washington, D.C.: The Advisory Board Company.

Clough, J. 2000. "Safety in the Delivery of Health Care." Paper presented at the National Heal Policy Forum, Washington, D.C., March 15.

Dwyer, K. 1998. "Medication-related Malpractice Claims." *Risk Management Foundation of the Harvard Medical Institutions Forum Report.* Boston: Harvard Medical Institutions.

Fink, J. 1983. "Legal Issues Surrounding the Number of Dosage Units Dispensed." *Drug Intelligence and Clinical Pharmacists* 17(10): 756–9.

Institute for Safe Medication Practices. 2000. *ISMP Medication Safety Self-Assessment.* Huntington, PA: ISMP.

Leape, L., A. Kabcenell, D. Berwick, and J. Roessner. 1998. *Reducing Adverse Drug Events.* Boston: Institute for Healthcare Improvement.

Leape, L., D.W. Bates, D.J. Cullen, J. Cooper, H.J. Demonaco, T. Gallivan, R. Hallisey, J. Ives, N. Laird, G. Laffell, R. Nemeskal, L.A. Petersen, K. Porter, D. Servi, B.F. Shea, S.D. Small, B.J. Sweitzer, T. Thompson, and M. Vander Vliet. 1995. "Systems Analysis of Adverse Drug Events." *Journal of the American Medical Association* 274(1): 35–43.

Harry, M., and R. Schroeder. 1999. *Six Sigma, The Breakthrough Management Strategy Revolutionizing the World's Top Corporations.* New York: Doubleday.

Moore, J. D. 1998. "Getting the Whole Story: The Way Medication Errors Are Reported Affects the Results." *Modern Healthcare* 18(51): 46.

U.S. House. Committee on Ways and Means. *Medical Liability: Impact on Hospital and Physician Costs Extends beyond Insurance.* 1995. Rept. AIMD-95-169.

CHAPTER SIX

Knowledge Management Loop to Match Staffing to Demand

Time is money.

—Benjamin Franklin

T HIS CHAPTER PROVIDES precise change concepts for recovering the costs associated with errors and other process inefficiencies that can be executed by the match staffing to demand team and other project leaders in their quality improvement work.

RECAPTURING LOST PRODUCTIVITY

As errors are reduced, more staff time becomes available. Using this chapter's change concepts, organizations can convert that free time into productivity gains. If the healthcare industry does not focus on recapturing the lost productivity and cost resulting from medical error reduction, it is doomed. An unsettling observation from the work of organizations leading the effort is that the concept of recapturing lost productivity is not on the radar screen. In fact, in more than one organization, productivity recapture was not only a foreign concept, but, once raised, was considered undesirable.

This is in stark contrast to the pioneering work of Deming and Juran as they coached manufacturing industries worldwide to improve quality and reduce costs. The automobile industry has seen a hundredfold improvement in defects per 100 cars while enjoying a tenfold improvement in productivity. Juran found that a distinct link between defects and lost productivity and the costs attributable to poor quality, as in healthcare, rested in a limited number of defect categories (Kanatsu 1990). Prior to the mastery of quality and error management by the American automobile industry, Japanese

	U.S.	Japan
Defects per 100 cars	33	24
Inventory	2 weeks	2 hours
Job classifications	9.5	2.9
Suppliers	509	170
Engineering done by suppliers	14 %	51 %
Production hours per car	31	16

manufacturers exceeded in every major category of quality and costs, as shown in Table 6.1 (Womack, Jones, and Roos 1990).

COST OF QUALITY

The heart of the quest for six sigma quality within the manufacturing and service industries resides not only in the gains in quality, but also in the major cost-competitive advantage enjoyed by producers with very low cost of quality (COQ) and cost of poor quality (COPQ). Inspection and inspector expense is simply not needed. These resources, at 33 percent of budget, can be redeployed to direct production or to lower the cost per unit of production.

A humorous story heard in many early quality training sessions makes the point. Apparently, an American company ordered some supplies from a Japanese company and part of its specifications were that only three defective parts per million would be accepted without penalty. Upon delivery, the American company found a small package next to a much larger package and an attached note that read: "The three defective parts you requested with your order are wrapped separately. Hope this pleases."

The assurance of quality and the COPQ are typically viewed by manufacturers as falling into one of four categories (Harry and Schroeder 1999):

1. internal failure costs;
2. external failure costs;
3. appraisal and inspection costs; and
4. prevention costs.

Internal failures comprise the largest category in both manufacturing and healthcare. This type of failure includes tasks and activities such as wasted effort and supplies, unnecessary complexity, rework, and work-arounds. During one cost reduction project, the consulting team discovered that the RNS, on average, were spending 24 percent of their time managing internal failures—calls to physicians or the pharmacy to clarify orders, trips to the pharmacy to retrieve medications, scavenger hunts for wheelchairs, or trips to central supply to pick up needed materials. Hidden inventories of supplies and linen on nurse units comprise another cost of poor quality associated with restocking processes that do not meet the needs of the nursing customers. Yet another form of internal failure in the medication management process is that of near misses, or those errors that are caught before the patient is affected.

External failures are internal failures that are not detected and mitigated and are experienced by one or more customers. In addition to the costs of internal failures, external failures carry the extra burden of warranty costs, malpractice indemnity awards and settlements, risk management research and analysis, and customer satisfaction recovery costs.

Appraisal and inspection costs (estimated in one organization to top 14 percent of total operating costs) consider each inspection point in every process (Caldwell 1994). For example, in a surgical process redesign a few years ago, we discovered that eight different inspection points existed to ensure the presence of lab, x-ray, and EKG reports in the patient's medical record prior to surgery. These eight inspections were being performed by three different professional groups, each one unknown to the other. After redesign, no inspections were required because the intake process included a forcing function that prevented errors from occurring. Appraisal and inspection costs also include the cost of quality assurance and of committee and staff costs for the detection, analysis, and corrective action of quality failures, such as nosocomial infections, surgical errors, medication errors, medical staff credentialing, falls, failures of communication, and clinical path variation.

Prevention costs include the traditional quality management functions of quality planning, improvement, and control; case management costs; risk management; infection control; training; and other costs incurred to ensure that quality levels are measured, detected, and corrected.

According to conventional wisdom, all but 50 percent of prevention and appraisal and inspection costs are the result of poor quality—hence, the reason that the drive for six sigma quality is such a critical strategy for manufacturers. Now that we have some appreciation for the types of costs that are required to ensure quality, let's look at the cost of quality at various sigma levels. Table 6.2 proves the point (Harry and Schroeder 1999).

Therefore, the typical U.S. IDN or medical center wastes approximately 33 percent of its resources on error detection, mitigation, and prevention. For every $100 million in operating budget, the CFO can be assured that

TABLE 6.2. COST COMPARISON FOR DIFFERENT SIGMA LEVELS

COST OF QUALITY

Sigma Level	Errors per Million Occurrences	Cost of Quality and Cost of Poor Quality (Internal Failure, External Failure, Appraisal and Inspection, Prevention)
2	308,537	uncompetitive
3	66,807	25–40 % of budget
4	6,210	15–25 % of budget
5	233	5–15 % of budget
6	3.4	world-class

about $33 million is devoted to the categories described above. Depending on whose estimate you choose—the medication management process, at 21 percent error rate according to Jhi, or Leape's estimate of 10 percent—at best falls into the 3 sigma class, consuming anywhere between 25 and 40 percent of the organization's budget (Advisory Board Company 1999).

The cost to ensure quality, or COQ and COPQ as quality professionals call these expense categories, consumes significant amounts of the typical organization's operating budget. Consider the effect in your organization when quality standards fail to achieve internal expectations. What happens when something goes wrong? A physician complains; an adverse drug event occurs; a surgical case starts 30 minutes late because the lab report is missing; a patient is delayed from going to imaging because a wheelchair cannot be found; it takes longer to prepare a patient room because there is no clean linen. All of these occurrences signify a deviation from defined quality standards of care.

The typical response to prevent repetition of a poor-quality event, such as those cases above, is to add one or more inspection steps. In some cases, this inspection is an addition to a staff member's current job, perhaps compounding negatively the quality of his or her direct-care tasks. In other cases, inspectors are added as full-time employees (FTES). Organizations that deploy case managers and care managers are, in fact, adding inspectors to ensure that their definition of quality, expressed in clinical paths or clinical guidelines, are met. Each of these professionals adds cost to the organization, rather than providing direct care. The effect of adding inspection and inspectors to an organization's COQ structure is shown in Figure 6.1.

FIGURE 6.1. COST OF QUALITY AT SIX SIGMA

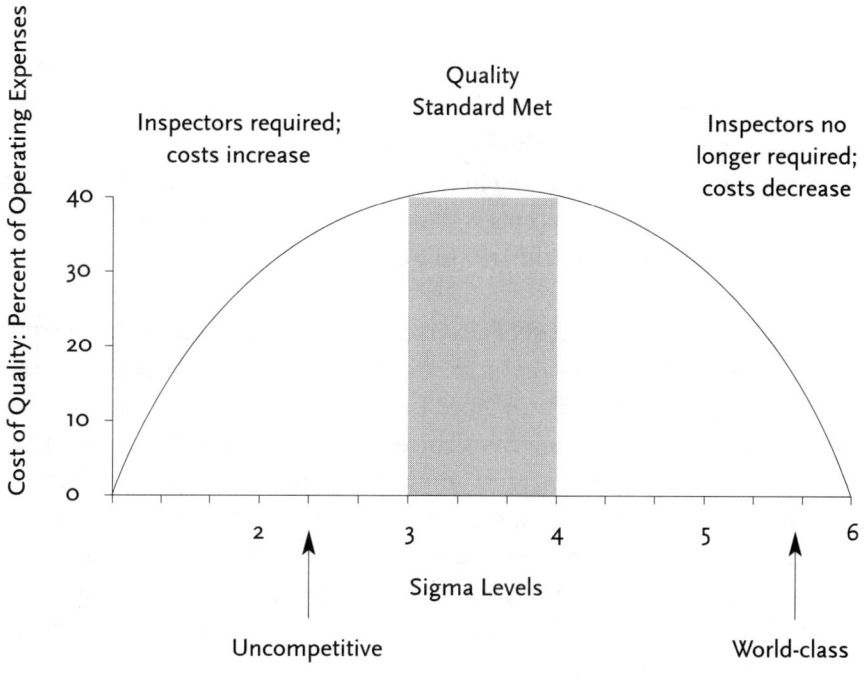

As Figure 6.1 so aptly illustrates, few (if any) manufacturing firms could price their products at levels acceptable to their customers at cost-of-quality levels below 2 sigma. The number of inspectors, the rework and work-arounds required to get products out the door, the warranty cost of returned products, and the cost of lost customers would simply be too high for these firms to sustain operations. Automobile plants, for example, have almost no rework and current levels continue to drop from their high of 25 percent of total worked hours in the 1980s (Womack, Jones, and Roos 1990).

Where did this rework occur? Womack analyzed U.S. automobile factories and discovered four categories of waste (Womack, Jones, and Roos 1990):

1. indirect workers;
2. excess inventory requiring ordering, reordering, accounting for multiple parts of virtually the same types from multiple suppliers;

3. work-arounds to make products, devices, and information systems work together that were not made to do so; and

4. dispirited workers who were frustrated and ashamed at their inability to do a good job.

Adequate research into the cost of medical and medication error in healthcare gives us pause, once again, to look to the successes in quality management in manufacturing. Although many argue that patient care and automobile production have nothing in common, it seems a strange paradox that the automobile industry accepts zero defects and six sigma achievement as a survival goal, but the healthcare industry seems to expect less for its patients.

One study placed the cost of adverse drug events and medication errors alone at $4.2 billion across the United States, or about $4,000 per discharge (Morelli 1997). A study of a 400-bed facility with 15,500 admissions annually found that the cost of adverse drug events and complications was $16.4 million, or about 2.5 percent of its annual budget (Advisory Board Company 1999). From the same study, examining just one subprocess—pharmacy productivity—the cost per 1,000 doses was $39.20. Or, looking at pharmacy cost management another way, 24 percent of the pharmacy budget is labor, so if a 10 percent medication error rate is present, 2.4 percent of pharmacy productivity is wasted effort (Advisory Board Company 1999).

How we view the relationship between medical errors, in general, and medication errors, in particular, is of critical importance to our potential for success. It has been troubling over the years to observe the differences in the quality and cost paradigm deployed by healthcare leaders compared to leaders of other industries. Healthcare leaders simply have failed to reach consensus on a reasonable definition of quality, globally and by diagnosis-related group (DRG) and functional department. Without a definition of quality, any equation becomes calculus and, hence, unmanageable. As illustrated below, the current debate of the past decade has been to solidify our agreement on the value delivered and we have made some (but inadequate) progress toward gains in quality, patient safety, and costs. Therefore, value, as perceived by the customer, is a function of the quality of services provided divided by the cost to provide those services.

$$\text{Value} = \frac{\textbf{Quality}}{\text{Cost/Resources}}$$

Where quality equals some ill-defined, elusive, locally determined measure, cost equals usually not one, but a number of different variables, such as cost per adjusted discharge, operating cost as a percent of net revenue, cost per covered life, and so on. In fairness, using acuity-adjusted costing methods, we have made great strides in the past several years in normalizing for comparative purposes.

Industry, on the other hand, tackled the issue of the quality and cost equation long ago by defining quality and cost strategically, in terms of customer expectations. Executive management realized that its role was to precisely define quality in terms of both features and acceptable error levels; it defined these thresholds through quality planning methods espoused by Juran and others. These expectations are expressed quite tightly. Defect levels are measured in terms of tolerances for variation from a customer-focused standard, such as plus or minus 0.03 millimeters from 16 millimeters or plus or minus two days from the promised delivery date. Then, executive management empowered the functional department managers by equipping them with training, coaching, tools, and measures to achieve these customer-driven goals at six sigma levels, or 3.4 occurrences per million.

Relate this management approach to healthcare. Healthcare executives, on average, have become increasingly removed from customers—the patients (and their proxies, physicians, and payers). The effect of this separation has been a lack of uniformity and consistency from facility to facility, patient care unit to patient care unit, and DRG to DRG in the definition of customer requirements for quality. The industry has not uniformly defined acceptable variations, such as in the number of minutes from the scheduled medication delivery time or in the percent of patients not on the DRG 209 clinical path prophylactic antibiotic protocol.

After executive management has defined the quality standard, it is possible for process owners to effectively manage for quality. The equation for quality then becomes:

$$\text{Quality} = \frac{\textbf{Processes (Work)}}{\text{Cost/Resources}}$$

In this equation, "quality" equals the predefined quality standard, "processes" means the number of steps required to achieve the quality standard, and "resources" refers to the cost of staff and supplies, including the cost of the inspectors (case managers, management, etc.) required to perform those processes.

In the management of medications on a given patient unit, on a critical care unit, in the emergency department, or in surgical services, the standard becomes the variation in terms of the number of minutes from scheduled administration time to the time between physician order and actual administration.

The equation, like all equations, equals a constant. For illustration, let's say the equation must always equal "1" or the equation is out of balance, as shown below:

$$\frac{\text{Processes (Work)}}{\text{Cost/Resources}} = 1$$

If we implement one of the change concepts from chapter 5 on a patient unit, for example, the effect has been to decrease steps in the work and, hence, to reduce the amount of staff time required to perform the work. The equation for quality on the patient unit is out of balance and no longer equals "1."

$$\frac{\text{Processes (Work)} \quad \downarrow}{\text{Cost/Resources}} = 1$$

There are only two ways to put the quality equation back into balance on the patient care unit. First, we can increase the number of steps staff are performing, by either importing tasks from another department or adding time and/or steps to other processes, such as patient teaching.

$$\frac{\text{Processes (Work)} \quad \downarrow \uparrow}{\text{Cost/Resources}} = 1$$

Or, we can decrease the number of staff hours budgeted for the patient care unit.

$$\frac{\text{Processes (Work)} \quad \downarrow}{\text{Cost/Resources} \quad \downarrow} = 1$$

In other words, every time the medication management team implements a change from the medication error reduction change concepts database discussed in chapter 5, staff time is saved because the time devoted to errors has been reduced. The quality equation remains out of balance until a corresponding and equal change is made by the match staffing to demand team in either the numerator or the denominator.

The effect of this unbalancing and rebalancing of the quality equation over time is to improve quality and decrease costs, as both Deming and Juran promised more than three decades ago.

This logic has been proven in healthcare as well. In one HMO, for example, physician panel size was increased from 1,956 patients per physician to 2,279 patients per physician, a remarkable 17 percent increase in productivity (Goldfield and Nash 1999). This was accomplished, in part, by rebalancing the quality equation so that office visits per physician increased from 330 per month to 370 per month. In another study, 26 hours of case manager clinical path inspection time was reduced by converting selected path steps into standing orders (Goldfield and Nash 1999).

ROLE OF THE MATCH STAFFING TO DEMAND TEAM

As discussed in chapter 4, the last step in step 3 of the 100-Day Plan, "Implement Idealized Design Change Concepts," is to recapture lost productivity and cost. The burden of this activity falls to the match staffing to demand creative idea team. As was illustrated in Figure 5.2, the intervention approach to reduce errors and regain lost productivity caused by those errors requires both the identification of the error and the upstream inspections that failed to catch the error, and then a system to prevent chronic occurrence of the error. Once errors are eradicated, productivity is recaptured because inspection steps that are no longer required can be eliminated. The secret to cost recovery is converting the time saved from inspection elimination to staffing reduction over time.

As also illustrated in chapter 5, after the locus of the error has been determined, it is then possible to move upstream and locate the precise subprocess and activity or task-level cause of the error. Using the medication error reduction change concepts database, the project leader can introduce changes that eliminate or dramatically reduce the potential for future recurrence. The final task of the medication errors team is to create the process analysis spreadsheet (as was shown in Table 4.1), from which the project leader can determine which downstream steps to eliminate.

After the medication error team leader has completed the spreadsheet and implemented the changes needed to eliminate and/or mitigate the effects of adverse drug events and medication errors, it is time to recapture the productivity and cost lost because of the previous errors. To accomplish this, the spreadsheet is handed over to the match staffing to demand team, who then can work to convert those changes, and others to support them, into recaptured lost productivity for ultimate improvement in both quality and costs.

Following this prioritization logic enables the IDN and/or medical center to optimize deployment of change concepts and the resources and energy devoted to medication error reduction.

As with the medication error reduction change concepts database, the match staffing to demand database is not static but, instead, requires revitalization from time to time as the project leader charters projects to implement the changes. Recall from chapters 4 and 5 that the database is created through the retention of a subject matter expert (SME) to work for several days on-site with the project leader and the facilitator and, in circumstances of significant resistance to change, directly with the key stakeholders.

Listed below is a set of change concepts that can be used to set the match staffing to demand team on the proper course, derived significantly from the work of Tom Nolan and IHI's breakthrough work in wait time reduction (Nolan et al. 1998). After several cycles of implementation, the project leader will want to engage the knowledge management loop, pulling in one or more SMEs in match staffing to demand to expand and enhance the database.

1. Match staffing to demand.
   - Predict demand through the use of run charts and staff observation reporting analysis, particularly for high-intensity tasks such as medication administration.
   - Plot demand (number of patients) on the same graph as staffing and make adjustments to mirror the two, rather than scheduling staff according to historical procedures.
2. Shape demand.
   - Avoid scheduling "schedulable" tasks during known busy periods (meal periods, meds time, etc.).
   - Overlap shifts for predictably busy periods and reduce staff during predictably slower periods.
   - Use nonstandard shift times and schedules.
   - Schedule unpredictable OR cases late in the day or in a designated room. (Do not emphasize efficiency in this room.)
3. Minimize handoffs.
   - Have the same staff perform multiple functions.
   - Train staff to perform tasks and answer questions—rather than their having to ask another staff member or supervisor to intervene and write procedures—to avoid delays from staff intervention lag time.
4. Eliminate inspection.
   - Examine all processes and redesign them to remove inspection steps.

5. Consolidate functions and job classifications.
   - Partner with other departments to share common functions and reduce required hours to perform these functions (i.e., EKG and OR share scheduling staffing; ED nurses perform EKGS on weekends to improve quality/speed of EKG performance while reducing on-call and callbacks).
   - Reframe original demand for individualized service into a large cluster of services.
   - Standardize OR suites to maximize their flexibility versus specialization.
6. Eliminate steps in every process (Caldwell 1998).
   - Construct COPQ spreadsheets, time/motion studies, and non-value-added (NVA) spreadsheets, and eliminate steps in the process that add no value to the desired outcome.
   - In the COPQ/NVA spreadsheets, classify steps as:
     -value-added (VA) steps that must be performed to achieve the aim of the process from the "customer's" viewpoint;
     -non-value-added (NVA) steps that are not required to achieve the aim of the process from the "customer's" viewpoint, such as waiting for other dependent processes, any rework, duplicate recording of any information, most inspection steps, rechecking, most redundant process steps; or
     -business-value-added (BVA) steps not required to achieve the aim of the process from the "customer's viewpoint," such as record keeping, medical record functions, admission information, most data collected for nonclinical departments, and productivity monitoring.
7. Automate routine processes.
   - Use comparative data to determine potential opportunity areas.
   - Use standard analysis software to determine staffing by shift, day, and season.
   - Use standard software to schedule staff.
   - Use handheld computers in preop testing.
   - Deploy medication management bedside devices to eliminate manual MARS (medical administration records) and unnecessary calls to physicians and the pharmacy.
8. Eliminate or mitigate errors and mistakes.
9. Do tasks in parallel.
   - Examine processes to potentially perform a sequential subprocess in parallel with another process.
   - Prepare for surgery while setting up instruments.

- Obtain patient information during wait times.
- Begin discharge teaching during the admit process.

10. Use multiple processes.
    - Rather than using a one-size-fits-all process, use multiple versions of the process, each tailored to the different needs of customers or users.
    - Use a separate process for ED patients with less serious conditions.
    - Use a separate process for ED patients with extremity injuries.

11. Move steps closer together.
    - Move radiography equipment next to units, or ED, with high demand.
    - Move outpatient surgery support to OPS area.
    - Move patient's chart to bedside.
    - Examine the work flow of processes and relocate needed materials to position them in the path of the process, rather than placing them randomly in the room.

12. Convert internal steps to external.
    - Convert tasks that are done as part of the process to tasks that are performed ahead of time or deferred until later.
    - Have standardized doses available ahead of time.
    - Move consultations from the ED to the inpatient setting.
    - Customize central supplies for particular physicians.

13. Eliminate things that are not used.
    - Reduce inventory of seldom-used supplies and drugs.

14. Identify and manage constraints.
    - Find and remove constraints and bottlenecks in the system.
    - Make all operating rooms available.
    - Free up ED exam rooms.
    - Examine cost-benefit of providing additional equipment or rooms if capital expenditure reduces cost of staff wait times.
    - Optimize surgery team utilization instead of OR suite utilization.

15. Use contingency plans.
    - Prepare backup or contingency plans to deal with unexpected delays.
    - Prepare a contingency plan for when a physician is called to the ED or the OR.
    - Cross-train staff to meet shifting demand.

ROLE OF THE HUMAN RESOURCES COUNCIL

In most settings, the match staffing to demand team will be able to decrease the number of positions authorized but unable to effect processes to actually achieve the new level of productivity. Therefore, another body is required—the human resources (HR) council.

The job of the HR council is to drive improvement made by the medication error and match staffing to demand teams to bottom-line savings. Although the tactics to achieve reductions are commonly known, from attrition to layoffs to automatic reassignment, staff reductions will not be achieved without the disciplined actions of an individual manager or team.

In summary, by experimenting with these match staffing to demand change concepts in the match staffing to demand team and the HR council, organizations can recover much of the cost associated with errors.

REFERENCES

Caldwell, C. (ed.). 1998. *The Handbook for Managing Change in Healthcare*. Milwaukee, WI: ASQ Quality Press, 265–302.

Caldwell, C. 1994. "Cost of Poor Quality Assessment, Baton Rouge General Medical Center." *Unpublished research*. Baton Rouge, LA.

Clinical Initiatives Center. 1999. *Prescription for Change: Toward a Higher Standard in Medication Management*. Washington, D.C.: The Advisory Board Company.

Goldfield, N., and D. Nash (eds.). 1999. *Managing Quality of Care in a Cost-focused Environment*. Tampa, FL: American College of Physician Executives, 85.

Kanatsu, T. 1990. *TQC for Accounting*. Cambridge, MA: Productivity Press.

Harry, M., and R. Schroeder. 1999. *Six Sigma, The Breakthrough Management Strategy Revolutionizing the World's Top Corporations*. New York: Doubleday.

Morelli, J. 1997. "The Anatomy of a Medication Error: Why RPhs Make Mistakes." *Drug Topics* 141(9): 52.

Nolan, T., M. Schall, D. Berwick, and J. Roessner. 1998. *Reducing Waits and Delays*. Boston: Institute for Health Improvement.

Womack, J., D. Jones, and D. Roos. 1990. *The Machine That Changed the World*. New York: Harper Perennial.

CHAPTER SEVEN

Closing the Gaps

The greatest value in the world is the difference between what we are and what we can become.

—Ben Herbster

T HIS FINAL CHAPTER is constructed to provide a ready reference for exploring the various structures, change concepts, and success factors covered in this book.

First, the reader is encouraged to complete an assessment of organizational accelerators from chapter 3, and, second, to focus on planning considerations for deployment of the four-step model as addressed in chapter 4. Finally, the reader is provided a self-assessment of the deployment of change concepts listed in chapters 5 and 6.

A workbook format of this chapter is also available at *www.ACHE.org /pubs/caldwork.html.* This workbook can be printed and copied for use in your organization and offers a valuable tool for you, your board, and your managers—anyone that can benefit from such an action-planning activity. Its framework is the combination of a self-assessment and a planning guide that executive teams, financial managers, clinical and operations managers, and physicians charged with reducing medication errors and their associated costs can use to implement the topics discussed in the preceding chapters.

SECTION I. PRESENCE OF ACCELERATORS

1. Think about each accelerator and, on a scale of 1 to 5, rate your organization's effective use of each accelerator to combat adverse drug events and medication errors. Section II solicits selection of key accelerators to be optimized in your organization.

- Engage a star performer.
- Build passion around a common aim—winning.
- Plan to win.
- Organize the game plan around team core competencies, not the other way around.
- Play as a team, not as a collection of talented people.
- Ensure constancy of leadership and team membership.
- Encourage a "We can do anything" mentality.
- Each member of the team, not just the coach, holds others accountable.
- Only the best performers get to play; all others are traded.
- Mistakes are not acceptable; work toward flawless execution.
- Practice, practice, practice.
- Superior performance is driven from an attraction theory rather than a punishment mind-set.
- Strive for constant improvement.
- Have a way to keep score.
- Constant and immediate feedback from the scoreboard.
- There are frequent time-outs and a halftime to assess mistakes and correct them.
- Speed of decisions and actions is critical.
- You can only do one thing in a basketball arena—play basketball; no distractions.

2. Think about and list those accelerators that deserve the most attention. Then, for each accelerator, plot potential action plans to optimize their use. Consider what barriers might prevent full optimization of the accelerator, and what countermeasures might be deployed to neutralize them. Are there other leaders you can enlist to focus on this accelerator?

Presence of Organizational Belief System

Look back at the table discussed in chapter 3 regarding the transformation of the organization's belief system from one in which errors are considered an unfortunate, but inevitable, result of complex systems to one that is intolerant of errors.

List up to seven beliefs present in your organization and the desired state.

Based on gaps between the current state and the desired state, record interventions that might effectively transform your current belief system to the desired state, and a likely executive sponsor.

SECTION II. DEPLOYING THE 100-DAY PLAN

STEP 1. GENERATE ORGANIZATIONAL WILL TO REDUCE ERRORS

The first step in the 100-Day Plan management method is to generate organizational will by mobilizing for strategy deployment. As discussed numerous times, any successful initiative requires planning, preparation, publication of a precise aim, establishment of measures, assignment of accountable executives, process owners and analysts, and resources. Three tasks drive the completion of this step. The organization must:

- establish an accountable executive and committee structure;
- redesign the infrastructure for speed; and
- deploy a balanced scorecard and use 100-day milestones tracking.

Establish an Accountable Executive and Committee Structure

Commit to the Initiative

Every critical program must be given a "name" so that all key stakeholders can relate to the objectives consistently. Therefore, the first step is to name the initiative and articulate its scope and boundaries. What names might be effective?

Appoint an Executive Change Agent

The successful change agent will possess certain critical characteristics. In your organization and culture, what are some of those critical characteristics? Which executives come to mind?

In most cases, for the first 6 to 12 months, outside coaching by an experienced consultant (in the case of an IDN, an executive from a sister organization) accelerates results.

Conduct an Evidence of Readiness Assessment

Readiness to change perhaps rivals presence of an underlying, supportive belief system as the most critical factor to address prior to progressing to step 2. An accurate, honest assessment helps to spot gaps before they create problems later on the in the 100-Day Plan implementation. Refer to chapter 4 for additional discussion regarding the purposes and uses of the Evidence of Readiness Assessment.

Build a Critical Mass of Champions

Certain key executives, board members, physicians, and managers immediately come to mind as strong champions. Who are they?

Certain key executives, board members, physicians, and managers immediately come to mind as likely detractors. Who are they?

Most often, the logic of detractors is not unreasonable nor is it based on misperceptions. Based on your knowledge of these individuals, what are some of the reasons for their beliefs?

Establish Policies That Ensure Accountability and Rewards and Recognition

On a scale of 1 to 5, how would you rank the effectiveness of potential approaches given your culture, past experiences with similar techniques, and availability of champions to manage the activity for the following?

- Storyboards
- Creative idea committee reviews
- Storyboard reviews
- CEO rounds
- Staff newsletters and news releases
- Good Idea Club
- Merit reviews
- Awards programs
- Other _____
- Other _____

Based on your assessment, which activities should be deployed? Who might be a potential leader?

State the Intent of the Initiative in Terms of the Organization's Mission, Vision, and Values

What thoughts do you have about incorporating this initiative into the fiber of the organization?

Estimate the Resources Required

- What resources, including capital for automation, consulting expertise, benchmarking visits, and library materials, are likely to be required (not dollars, but deliverables)?
- Every successful initiative requires time, a scare resource in most orga-

nizations. What key individuals must be involved, and how many hours per week must be freed up? Include specific individuals, such as pharmacy chief, and groups of managers, such as nursing unit managers.

- What can be done to make this time available? Include redeployment of the individual's existing projects to others, delay of noncritical projects, or engagement of outside consultants to complete critical projects that cannot be delayed.

Deploy a Communication Plan

- Which constituency groups are important to consider?
- What existing communication vehicles are currently in existence to convey critical messages and progress?
- Who should be assigned to complete the communication plan and present recommendations?

Milestone date present _____

Redesign the Infrastructure for Speed

Charter the Creative Idea Committee

Frequently, executives and staff end up on committees of this type by default because everyone with any possible connection to any potential solution is tapped to serve. The ideal selection method is to (1) determine the critical criteria and executive-level support required to drive medication error reduction; and (2) appoint logical individuals. Those having a moderate or slight influence on potential solutions, such as the CFO or CIO, should be appointed as ex officio or ad hoc members (generally appreciated because of other pressing executive priorities). However, it is usually better to follow an inclusive, rather than an exclusive, approach and include any executive with a passion for the initiative. Based on these considerations, what criteria and support requirements exist for an aggressive medication error reduction program to flourish?

The creative idea committee is chaired by the executive change agent and supported by other leaders in the organization. What candidates come to mind as potential committee members? As the potential chair?

Appoint a Facilitator to Manage the Creative Idea Committee

The successful facilitator will possess certain critical characteristics. In your organization and culture, what are some of those critical characteristics?

Most often, facilitator candidates come from quality management and management engineering. What candidates come to mind?

In most cases, for the first 6 to 12 months, coaching by an outside consultant (in the case of an IDN, a facilitator from a sister organization) with experience in medication error reduction will accelerate results.

Charter Creative Idea Teams

Refer to Figure 4.5, Creative Idea Team Structure, and the related discussion for suggestions about team structure and process effects.

Based on your current situation, who are the most likely members of creative idea teams? Who are the potential leaders? Write a tentative or draft goal for each of the following creative idea teams (e.g., to reduce adverse drug events in surgical processes by 30 percent in 18 months).

- Surgical Errors Team
- Medication Errors Team
- Women's Healthcare Errors Team
- Critical Care Errors Team
- Reporting and Analysis Group

Redesign All Decision Processes for Speed

During the kickoff of the medication error reduction initiative, or at some other convenient gathering, assemble creative idea team members for a three-hour decision-making process redesign session. Break members into different groups, and ask them to brainstorm and nominally group barriers to speedy decisions. Their list will most likely be complete and comprehensive. After report-outs by each table, select the top four to five barriers and reassign team members to tables designated to brainstorm creative solutions to each identified barrier. Again, conduct report-outs. At the conclusion of this activity, the reporting and analysis group should construct leading barriers and potential solutions for the creative idea committee to implement.

Train Staff in the Core Competencies Required to Implement Idealized Design Change Concepts

Based on the discussion in chapter 4, what are possible core competencies that might be strengthened with focused training and mentoring? Also list potential sources, both internal and external, for training.

Deploy 100-Day Milestones Tracking and Balanced Scorecard

Establish Measurement and Milestone Reporting Process

List potential balanced scorecard measures, including no more than one measure for medication error reduction. What is the frequency (i.e. monthly or quarterly)? What are the potential sources?

STEP 2. CONDUCT A COMPARATIVE DATA AND GAP ANALYSIS

The outcome of this step is the publication of three-year objectives and one-year goals for each creative idea team. The teams examine available data to determine their gaps from peer comparisons, if reasonably available, or internal historical data, if comparisons are absent.

Set Targets Using Comparative Data

From the starting point of these suggested performance measures for the medication errors team, and adding any that are appropriate for your IDN or enterprise, set draft stretch goals to discuss with your colleagues. Line through the suggested goals below that are not applicable to your IDN or medical center. Remember that in a culture of "stretch," failure to achieve stretch does not signify a punishable event but, rather, a charter for another round of continuous performance activity on the road to world-class quality.

Charter Projects Aligned to Targets

As discussed in chapter 4, step 2 of the 100-Day Plan method requires that projects be chartered in order to achieve the stretch goal. During the first and second sessions, the team should envision this future state. Some team members will embrace this world-class state with vigor; others will be overcome by the fear of failure. It is vital to ultimate success that all team members share a vision of the future state and the changes that will be required. Several steps will aid this process:

1. Re-record the vision.
2. Brainstorm characteristics of the current state of the medication management system, using a cause-and-effect diagram approach to stimulate characteristics for all key components of the system.

Medication Errors Team Goal Setting

Goal	Comparative Benchmark or Budget Performance	Nonstretch Potential Three-Year Goal	Potential Stretch Three-Year Goal (20 to 30% higher)	Potential One-Year Stretch Goal (recommend 50% of three-year stretch)
Medication errors per adjusted discharge				
Monthly manager activity results score				
Operating cost per adjusted discharge				
FTES per adjusted occupied bed				
Adverse events per discharge				
Prescribing errors per prescription				
Ordering errors per prescription				
Fulfillment errors per prescription				
Administration error per prescription				
Medication process cost per discharge (incl. staff cost) (or the proxy pharmacy department total cost and all patient care units total cost)				
Patient care hours per patient day				
Pharmacy cost per prescription				
Other				

A. People in the system (caregivers, management and executive staff, physicians, support staff). What are the current state characteristics? What are the future state characteristics?

B. What are the processes (procedures, policies, guidelines, clinical paths, formulary, etc.)?

C. What are the systems (IT, robotics, medical records, admitting, staff scheduling, etc.)?

D. Environment (managed care and Medicare requirements, regulatory requirements, etc.)?

E. Beliefs about adverse drug events and medication errors and the medication management process?

F. Other critical categories

3. Can you think of a one- to three-sentence descriptor of the future state, world-class medication management process?

Set Targets Using Comparative Data for Both Cost and Speed

1. Assess your current effectiveness in using comparative data to set targets and chartering projects aligned to organizational priorities. Using a 1–5 scale, with "1" indicating a problem area and "5" indicating strong presence of this leverage factor throughout the organization, score yourself below.

2. For each factor scoring less than "4," list the causes for suboptimal performance, and,

3. Consider chartering a team to improve your score over the next few months.

Score yourself (1 to 5):

- Do not permit delay while searching for the "perfect" data or source of data.
- Avoid collecting data on every conceivable control variable.
- Set true stretch goals, not simply what is conceivable at the moment.
- Be diligent in constructing project milestone dates and in using the 100-Day Plan Project Planner. This assures the Medication Error Team, and, ultimately the Creative Idea Team, stays on track and that the current position relative to the goal is known at critical times during the initiative.
- The Match Staffing to Demand Team's ability to creatively recapture lost productivity regained by patient safety teams into true, bottom-line benefits to the organization's customers.

STEP 3. IMPLEMENT IDEALIZED DESIGN CHANGE CONCEPTS

From chapter 4, outlining step 3, recall the following tasks:

- Search or create change concepts databases in the Knowledge Management Loop.
- Implement 30-day cycle Aim-Measure- PDSA ramps.
- Track to assure projects stay on track.

1. Assess your current effectiveness at execution, using a 1–5 scale, with "1" indicating a problem area and "5" indicating strong presence of this leverage factor throughout the organization, score yourself below.
2. For each factor scoring less than "4," list the causes for suboptimal performance, and,
3. Consider chartering a team to improve your score over the next few months.

Rate performance in each of the following critical success factors (1 to 5):

- Resist straying from the original aim
- Set aggressive stretch goals
- Avoid too many or ineffective measures
- Do not wait for Information Systems to provide the measure; use sampling when manual collection is required
- To ensure momentum, craft plans for the next two to three cycles
- Select changes that are acceptable to the majority
- Strive to learn and improve the process after each cycle
- If it can't be tested in the next thirty days, move on to the next idea
- Steal shamelessly from others
- Engage defined activity to recapture lost productivity and cost to convert error reduction into bottom-line impact

STEP 4. HOLD THE GAINS

1. Assess your current effectiveness at holding the gains, using a 1–5 scale, with "1" indicating a problem area and "5" indicating strong presence of this leverage factor throughout the organization, score yourself below.
2. For each factor scoring less than "4," list the causes for suboptimal performance, and,

3. Consider chartering a team to improve your score over the next few months.

Rate performance in each of the following activities (1 to 5):

- Adjust Balanced Scorecard thresholds to accommodate the new level of performance.
- Auditing, at the department level, to assure gains are held.
- Conduct a review of manager audit techniques at a monthly manager meeting so that learning of best practices occurs.

SECTION III. EFFECTIVE DEPLOYMENT OF MEDICATION ERROR CHANGE CONCEPTS

As discussed in chapter 5, an assessment of the optimization of known change concepts may be a good way to get started and/or reenergized. The assessment below can be used to jump-start this process.

For the following list, rank your current optimization of change concepts. Use the Institute for Healthcare Improvement Breakthrough scale (below). What is your total score? Your average score? Upon completion of the scoring, list those change concepts with a low score and consider how you might optimize the potential offered by adopting these change concepts. Consider marking your calendar six months from the date of the first assessment and repeat the assessment process to determine the organization's rate of execution.

1 = Nonstarter, no activity. The organization has engaged limited, if any, effort in the change concepts listed.

2 = Activity, but no strategic change. The organization has actively studied and discussed the change concepts but has not changed any practices, or the change concepts that have been implemented have produced no reduction in errors and/or costs.

3 = Activity with improvement in medication errors, but no recovery of costs associated with errors. The organization has reduced medication errors, but no activities have recovered costs.

4 = Activity, medical error reduction with one-time cost recovery. The organization has implemented many of the change concepts listed and has collected data demonstrating close to 100 percent achievement of stated goals

of the projects. Moreover, it has executed change concepts to recover one-time costs such as inventory reductions (e.g., has achieved a goal for reducing administration errors but has not executed any change concepts to increase productivity of staff previously busy correcting these errors).

5 = Activity, medical error reduction with sustainable cost recovery. The organization has implemented virtually all change concepts in the area listed and has data to suggest leading-edge performance in this area. Moreover, it has recovered much of the associated costs of these errors (e.g., has achieved a goal of 50 percent reduction in adverse drug events in a critical care unit and has recaptured the saved time by assigning one more patient to each critical care nurse while maintaining the number of minutes per patient).

Change Concept

1. Reduce reliance on memory using techniques such as:
   - drug–drug interaction checking systems;
   - computerized order entry;
   - widely used guided-dose algorithms;
   - laminated dosing cards to help remember tasks;
   - bar coding to match drug bar code to patient wristband bar code;
   - computerized patient information (including allergy information); and
   - computerized drug dispensing, and timers or alarms.
2. Simplify processes by:
   - eliminating order transcription;
   - limiting choice of available drugs in pharmacy;
   - limiting the choices of dosage strengths and concentration for each drug (use a maximum of 2);
   - maintaining inventory of frequently used prepared drugs, rather than preparing such drugs to order;
   - limiting the number of times per day that drugs are administrated, mix IVs in the pharmacy; and
   - using a single record entry for medications, automating dispensing on the unit.
3. Standardize by:
   - standardizing prescribing conventions (use no abbreviations) -use "units" vs. "u"; use leading zero [0.5 not 5] but avoid trailing zero [5 not 5.0], -use generic names, -use metric system only, -do not use Q or q;

- using protocols for complex medication administration (heparin, insulin, chemotherapy);
- limiting the number of standard doses of medication;
- standardizing times of drug administration;
- storing medications in the same place in every medication room;
- standardizing packaging and labeling for all medications (make "like" drugs look alike and different drugs that are different); and
- using standard equipment (e.g., one kind of pump).

4. Use constraints and forcing functions by:
   - using pharmacy computers that will not fill any orders unless allergy information and patient weight and height are entered;
   - adding special luer-locks to syringes and indwelling lines that have to match before fluid can be infused, thus preventing personnel from infusing non-iv solutions into ivs, central lines, or intrathecal lines;
   - using computerized order with range checks on doses to prevent completion of an order until the dose specified is in a safe range for the medication and patient; and
   - removing concentrated potassium chloride solutions from floor stock, thus preventing accidental rapid iv infusion of a concentrated solution.

5. Use protocols and checklists wisely by:
   - avoiding statements that contain negatives (e.g., "Check to see that the light is off" is better than "Check to see that the light is not on");
   - making instructions agree with the most likely state of the system (so that a yes is the usual response); and
   - ensuring that everyone has agreed on the protocol or checklist regularly to understand what exceptions may require revision of the protocol or checklist.

6. Improve access to information by:
   - having a pharmacist available on the nursing units and at rounds;
   - using computerized order-entry systems;
   - using computerized patient information;
   - using computerized laboratory data to immediately alert clinicians about abnormal lab values;
   - placing lab reports and medication records at the bedside;
   - placing protocols and ordering information on the patient's chart and in the medication room where they are easily accessible;
   - color-coding wristbands for patients with allergies;
   - providing each patient with allergies with a list of his or her medications, doses, and times;

- tracking errors or near misses and reporting them to staff on a weekly basis; and
- accelerating lab turnaround times for blood coagulation tests (partial thromboplastic time, or PTTs) and blood sugar tests.

7. Decrease reliance on vigilance by:
   - using automatic drug dose checking in high-risk situations;
   - using double-checks for doses of narcotics, insulin, heparin, chemotherapy, and other lethal drugs;
   - having the pharmacist monitor highly toxic drugs on a daily basis;
   - using checklists and standardizing their use at regular intervals (e.g., checking temperature every 15 minutes for blood products);
   - using electronic monitors that signal an alarm when parameters are exceeded, but using them carefully (they do not substitute for attention);
   - limiting long shifts for physicians, nurses, and pharmacists; and
   - rotating staff who are performing repetitive functions.

8. Reduce handoffs by:
   - providing ready-to-administer products; reducing transcription of medical orders;
   - using unit dosing systems, having a pharmacist participate in rounds;
   - using automated point-of-care drug delivery systems:
   - using a computerized prescriber for order entry; and
   - using a satellite pharmacy.

9. Decrease multiple entry by:
   - using a computerized prescriber order entry that automatically transmits the physician's order to both the pharmacy and the nursing station; and
   - having the pharmacy generate a computerized medication administration record.

10. Differentiate—eliminate look-alikes and sound-alikes by:
    - repackaging or relabeling look-alike medications to differentiate them;
    - storing similar-looking medications in separate places;
    - alerting staff and posting information on sound-alike medications (some organizations avoid sound-alikes by using the brand name for one medication and the generic name for the other); and
    - avoiding stocking look-alike packages.

11. Automate carefully with techniques such as:
    - computerized order-entry systems with range checks and override capacity;

- robotic dispensing systems in the pharmacy;
- staff training to double-check the automation regularly, thus keeping skill levels high and reinforcing the idea that all systems must be monitored; and
- bar code technology to identify drugs.

12. Optimize the work environment for safety by:
- keeping workloads within an acceptable range;
- reducing unnecessary time pressure in any phase of the medication system;
- avoiding double shifts, accommodating diurnal sleep rhythms;
- adjusting the physician environment to increase light, decrease noise, and decrease clutter;
- keeping critical equipment available, in good repair, and stored in a uniform manner; and
- reducing distractions.

13. Increase immediate feedback by:
- using equipment that not only indicates there is a problem but also shows where the problem is;
- monitoring the effectiveness of protocols instituted and providing information to all staff demonstrating the effectiveness of protocols; and
- making staff aware of responses to reported errors.

14. Train for teamwork by:
- training leaders in a nonauthoritarian style of management; and training workers to function as a team;
- training workers to be interdependent as well as independent;
- training for safety, emphasizing potential hazards and methods to avoid them; and
- creating stable teams to work with high-hazard substances.

15. Drive out fear by:
- publicly rewarding reports of error (e.g., with release time or a thank-you from the CEO);
- establishing safe havens for error reporting (e.g., granting immunity from punishment);
- establishing confidential reporting of errors;
- making error reporting easy (e.g., using simple forms);
- conducting regular small group discussions of "errors waiting to happen";
- collecting and disseminating information on common errors in the organization (e.g., feedback information to clinicians);
- displaying run charts to show the effects of error reduction efforts, such as compliance with protocols, reduction of

nonstandard orders, or automatic dose reduction for the elderly; and

- displaying run charts to show increased reporting of errors.

16. Obtain leadership commitment by:
    - decreasing competition and increasing cooperation among staff;
    - creating interdisciplinary teams;
    - publicly thanking staff for reports of errors; and
    - committing resources to make the environment safe, establishing effective error reporting systems, improving work conditions, and providing time to analyze errors.

17. Improve direct communication by:
    - training all staff to avoid indirect and mitigated communication;
    - repeating verbal orders verbatim;
    - role-playing direct communication and methods for dealing with authoritarian style; and
    - providing feedback (including feedback in videotape format) about indirect and mitigated communication.

SECTION IV. EFFECTIVE DEPLOYMENT OF MATCH STAFFING TO DEMAND CHANGE CONCEPTS

As in the previous exercise, rank your current optimization of change concepts using the Institute for Healthcare Improvement Breakthrough scale (below). What is your total score? Your average score? Upon completion of the scoring, list those change concepts with a low score and consider how you might optimize the potential offered by adopting these change concepts. Consider marking your calendar six months from the date of the first assessment and repeat the assessment process to determine the organization's rate of execution.

1 = Nonstarter, no activity. The organization has engaged limited, if any, effort in the change concepts listed.

2 = Activity, but no strategic results. The organization has actively studied and discussed the change concepts but has not changed any practices.

3 = Activity, with some timesaving. The organization has implemented some of the areas mentioned and has collected evidence that the change saved staff time but has not yet recaptured lost productivity through staffing changes.

4 = Activity, with one-time cost recovery. The organization has implemented many of the change concepts listed and has collected data demonstrating one-time savings (such as inventory reduction).

5 = Activity, with sustainable cost recovery. The organization has implemented virtually all change concepts in the area listed and has data to suggest leading-edge performance in this area.

Change Concept

1. Match staffing to demand.
   - Predict demand through the use of run charts and staff observation reporting analysis, particularly for high-intensity tasks such as medication administration.
   - Plot demand (number of patients) on the same graph as staffing and make adjustments to mirror the two, as opposed to scheduling staff according to historical procedures.
2. Shape demand.
   - Avoid scheduling "schedulable" tasks during known busy periods (meal periods, meds time).
   - Overlap shifts for predictably busy periods and reduce staff during predictably slower periods.
   - Use nonstandard shift times and schedules.
   - Schedule unpredictable OR cases late in the day or in a designated room. (Do not emphasize efficiency in this room.)
3. Minimize handoffs.
   - Have the same staff perform multiple functions.
   - Train staff to perform tasks, answer questions versus having to ask for another staffperson or supervisor to intervene and write procedures in order to avoid delays because of staff intervention lag time.
4. Eliminate inspection.
   - Examine all processes and redesign them to remove inspection steps.
5. Consolidate functions, job classifications.
   - Partner with other departments to share common functions, reducing required hours to perform them (e.g., EKG and OR share scheduling staffing; ED nurses performing EKGs on weekends to improve quality/speed of EKG performance while reducing on-call, callbacks).
   - Reframe original demand for individualized service into a large cluster of services.

- Standardize OR suites to maximize their flexibility rather than specialization.

6. Eliminate steps in every process (Caldwell 1998).
   - Construct COPQ spreadsheets, time/motion studies, and non-value-added spreadsheets, and eliminate steps in the process that add no value to the desired outcome.

7. Automate routine processes.
   - Use comparative data to determine potential opportunity areas.
   - Use standard analysis software to determine staffing by shift, by day, by season.
   - Use standard software to schedule staff.
   - Use handheld computers in preop testing.
   - Deploy medication management bedside devices to eliminate manual MARS, unnecessary calls to physicians and pharmacy.

8. Eliminate, mitigate errors, mistakes.
   - Do tasks in parallel.
   - Examine processes to potentially perform a sequential subprocess in parallel with another process.
   - Prepare for surgery while setting up instruments.
   - Obtain patient information during wait times.
   - Begin discharge teaching during the admit process.

9. Use multiple processes.
   - Rather than using a one-size-fits-all process, use multiple versions of the process, each tailored to the different needs of customers or users.
   - Use a separate process for ED patients with less serious conditions.
   - Use a separate process for ED patients with extremity injuries.

10. Move steps closer together.
   - Move radiography equipment next to units, or ED, with high demand.
   - Move outpatient surgery support to OPS area.
   - Move patient's chart to bedside.
   - Examine the work flow of processes and relocate needed materials to position them in the path of the process, rather than being placed randomly in the room.

11. Convert internal steps to external.
   - Convert tasks that are done as part of the process to tasks that are performed ahead of time or deferred until later.
   - Have standardized doses available ahead of time.
   - Move consultations from the ED to the inpatient setting.
   - Customize central supplies for particular physicians.

12. Eliminate things not used.
    - Reduce inventory of seldom-used supplies and drugs.
13. Identify and manage constraints.
    - Find and remove constraints and bottlenecks in the system.
    - Make all operating rooms available.
    - Free up ED exam rooms.
    - Examine cost-benefit of providing additional equipment, rooms, if capital expenditure reduces cost of staff wait times.
    - Optimize surgery team utilization rather than OR suite utilization.
14. Use contingency plans.
    - Prepare backup or contingency plans to deal with unexpected delays.
    - Prepare a contingency plan for when a physician is called to ED or OR.
    - Cross-train staff to meet shifting demand.

REFERENCE

Caldwell, C. (ed.). 1998. *The Handbook for Managing Change in Healthcare*. Milwaukee, WI: ASQ Quality Press, 265–302.

Index

About the Authors

CHIP CALDWELL, FACHE

Chip Caldwell is the president of Chip Caldwell & Associates, specializing in strategic deployment of clinical and systems quality improvement, 6 sigma, and cost reduction initiatives in medical centers, extended care facilities, integrated health systems, and health plans. Mr. Caldwell's previous positions include senior vice president of Premier Performance Services; health industry executive of Juran Institute; president of the HCA Atlanta health system; and president and CEO of HCA West Paces Medical Center in Atlanta. He served on the Baldrige Foundation Board Support Team in 1999 and 2000 and was the only healthcare representative on the U.S. Quality Council in 2000.

He has trained over 10,000 personnel in organizations including IBM, Scripps Health System, Veterans' Administration, PruCare, Kaiser, the U.S. Navy, and the Sisters of Mercy Health System. He was selected by the European Organization for Quality to head the European Demonstration Project in December 1994.

Mr. Caldwell has keynoted seminars for JCAHO, AHA, National Patient Safety Summit, EBM Solutions, Harvard's Institute for Healthcare Improvement, Australia Minister of Health Conference, National Healthcare Forum, Ontario Hospital Association, Group Health Association of America and Massachusetts Hospital Association. His other books include *Mentoring Strategic Change in Health Care: An Action Guide* (ASQC) and *The Handbook for Managing Change in Healthcare* (ASQC).

CHARLES R. DENHAM, M.D.

Dr. Charles Denham is CEO of HCC Corporation. Launched in 1983, it has led, developed, or supported over 300 product development teams in over 50 product categories including pharmaceutical, medical, and surgical devices, and software. With Premier and major supplier companies, Dr. Denham founded the Premier Innovation Institute, which is dedicated to equip providers and suppliers with solutions to meet their innovation adoption and market penetration challenges.

Dr Denham undertook specialty training at the Baylor College of Medicine and practiced as a radiation oncologist for 12 years. He has been an associate professor of biomedical engineering at the University of Texas since 1983 and has taught innovation transfer at a number of medical and business schools. In 1983 he founded the Texas Medical Institute of Technology, a nonprofit research foundation dedicated to bridging the gap between basic science innovation and clinical utilization.

The son of a NASA computer scientist, Dr. Denham grew up in the shadow of the Apollo program. His interest in the application of aviation methods to medicine and patient safety has intensified throughout his career as a radiation oncologist, teacher, and leader in healthcare innovation transfer. In the 1980's as the owner of an aircraft manufacturing company, his team was simultaneously leading aircraft accident and hospital adverse event investigations. These parallel experiences demonstrated the great learning opportunity aviation provides to healthcare.